Wishing you the best of living your recovery!
Mary Moeller

Fibromyalgia Cookbook

A Daily Guide to Becoming Healthy Again

MARY MOELLER

Published by: Fibromyalgia Solutions 305 East Ninth Street Kearney, Missouri 64060

Illustrations by Simon Moeller

Notice to Reader

Consult with your doctor before embarking on this or any other nutritional or exercise program. The information contained within this workbook is designed for persons who are suffering from fibromyalgia. It is in no way intended as a substitute for medical counseling. The creators of this workbook disclaim any liability for loss in connection with the information expressed herein.

Acknowledgments

I would like to thank the following people for their help:

Dr. Randy Dierenfield for his help and patience in working with me to overcome the challenge of fibromyalgia.

Dr. Brian Kelling for his help and support during my healing process.

Dr. Dawn Leibrandt for the treatments she gave me to keep me going.

Dr. William Shaw for his research to help all of us afflicted with FMS.

Simon Moeller for his expertise and work in helping to write this book.

Kelly Moeller for working with me to overcome her symptoms.

Karl Moeller for his love, and for supporting me during many years of illness. It was his love that kept me going during those dark years when I felt there was no hope of ever feeling well again, and it is his love and support today that is helping me to help others learn what they can do to feel well again.

Table of Contents

Fibromyalgia   7

A Few More Thoughts   9

Using and Completing the Workbook   9

Sleep Aids   137

Pain Aids   139

Supplements   141

Stretching Exercises   141

Acupressure Points   148

Appendix   155

ILLUSTRATIONS

Stretching Exercises   143

Acupressure Points   149

Fibromyalgia

For those of us with fibromyalgia (FMS), life as we once knew it has changed drastically. We know and understand all too well the symptoms and complaints we share, as well as the lifestyle changes that have taken place since the onset of our symptoms. For me the symptoms started almost 35 years ago, long before the term "fibromyalgia" was in my physicians vocabulary. As with most of us, the symptoms seemed to gradually consume every part of my being. However, it wasn't until my daughter was diagnosed with FMS that I became serious about trying to combat the effects of this illness. Many mornings upon waking, I had mentioned to my husband , that this life may not be worth living if I had to live the rest of it in the extreme pain and with the overwhelming symptoms of fibromyalgia. It was especially disturbing to imagine my then 9 year old daughter possibly developing those same feelings. So, with my daughter's and my own well being as a motivator, I set out on a long, challenging, and yes, rewarding journey to wellness.

Today my daughter and I share predominately symptom free, healthful lives. I am now able to do at 45 years of age, more than I was able to do at 30 years of age, and I feel like a "million dollars" most of the time. My daughter is symptom free at age 14, is as active and energetic as any other 14-year-old. It hasn't been easy, there were no "magic pills" to take to make the symptoms go away. There were, however many result oriented steps which were discovered, which led to a natural healthful control of the many symptoms of fibromyalgia. I will share those steps with you, through the use of a four-month plan which is result oriented. So, as you learn, you also can see the results in our own body.

Overcoming the symptoms of FMS does not happen overnight. It took almost a year to feel completely well again. Kelly took a little less time, possibly because we caught it shortly after she started having symptoms. And getting better requires a complete lifestyle change encompassing our diets, exercise, sleep habits and even how we interact with family and friends. One can expect anywhere from one to three months of work on these changes before any positive effects can be seen in the symptoms. Those who have been able to overcome the FMS challenge have not done so overnight, it takes time, patience and perseverance. But you can feel better, and once you have achieved that goal, you will feel that it has been worth every effort you have made.

Imagine having the energy to play that tennis game, ride your bike, keep your house clean, go to that party. Or maybe, as with others, your goal may be to be able to comfortably hold your newborn baby. You can do it! Look at this as a long term project which you will work on each and every day, one day at a time. Set a year from now as your goal to feel better. As the year passes by, you will notice you are doing more and more. As days turn into months, each month will show the improvements you are making. When you get frustrated and tired of trying, read back through your workbook and take note of the things that have improved from one week to another.

After three months, Jan, a client I was working with, was feeling she had not gained anything since starting the program. In looking back through the records, she was now staying up 8-10 hours a day instead of just one to three hours when she had first started the program. She was now exercising between 30 and 60 minutes, and when she had started she was unable to exercise due to the extreme fatigue and pain. Another lady, after looking back at her workbook, saw that after four months she was able to once again drive her car and get her own groceries. And she was able to exercise and do light yard work for periods lasting between one to three hours.

The changes take place very gradually. As many of the professionals I have worked with reminded me while I was on the road to recovery, "You didn't get this overnight, and you won't be able to overcome it overnight." It has taken months or years to acquire the symptoms of FMS, so it will take some time for the body to heal.

This workbook is designed to help you make the lifestyle changes necessary to begin the healing process. It covers the first 120 days, and will help you make the basic changes needed to begin feeling better. Once you have covered approximately four months of lifestyle changes, you will have what you need to continue your journey to feeling and keeping healthy.

Everything Kelly and I have done to get better has been accomplished without the aid of prescription medication. This program is in no way meant to replace your medical treatment, or regular trips to your physician. Over time, while continuing consultations with your physician, you may find than trips to the doctor will become less frequent. There is a section in the back of the book which covers natural remedies for pain control, sleep disturbances, muscle relaxation and muscle stretching exercises. Refer to this section of the workbook whenever you need helpful hints in these areas. And remember, always consult with you physician or health professional before embarking on this journey to health!

It is very important to follow this workbook on a daily basis to feel better. Take it with you as your daily planner so you will be able to keep records on a regular basis. Keeping it near your side will also help you avoid some of the "no-nos" which could throw you off track, along with giving you encouragement to keep trying. If you slip periodically, that's okay. Start again the next day. Remember you didn't get this illness overnight, it may take awhile to feel better, so if you slip up, you always have tomorrow to begin again. This may be one of the hardest challenges you have had to overcome, together we can do it. You will be so happy you did and I will be happy for you!

There are many different ideas as to why FMS makes it debut in the health of its victims. If you have done any research on your own, you probably have some of your own thoughts in this matter. There is the theory that an overgrowth of yeast within a person's system can be a cause for many of the symptoms of FMS. Another thought is that the immune system has been impaired in some way, possibly by injury, which can cause symptoms as well as the malabsorption of vitamins and minerals consumed by the victim. Still another theory is a possible build-up of toxins within our systems, which some of us are unable to discard. These toxins eventually manifest as fibromyalgia or chronic fatigue syndrome. The list goes on and on.

Whatever the theory, I do know that the need for supplements is very real. For my daughter and myself, many supplements seemed to have little or no effect on us. I pay very close attention as to how Kelly and I feel after taking a vitamin supplement, especially for the first couple of weeks. We should notice increased energy, as well as lessened pain. Also, cognitive thinking and memory should improve markedly after about three to five weeks of consumption. In addition, I feel is has been important to take both a nutritional supplement (one which gives us an increase in nutritional value as if we were eating all the fruits and vegetables we could possibly put into our bodies), and a mineral supplement. The mineral supplements should contain as many of the essential minerals necessary for healthy bodies as is humanly possible to stick into a bottle. I feel our bodies have done better on liquid or capsule forms than on pill forms of supplements. You will find additional information on supplements in the back of this workbook.

Before you begin to use the workbook, fill out the Health Evaluation Form as a guide to how you are feeling at this time. Every month there will be another Health Evaluation Form (or HEF) to fill out so you can keep track of your own progress.

It was not uncommon for Kelly and I to have a couple of good days and then seem to fall back into a relapse. Know that the frequency of your relapses will decrease with time. At times you may feel like you aren't improving, but that is all part of the healing cycle, especially if your FMS is part of a yeast overgrowth. Keep on the schedule and continue each day working to accomplish the goals in the workbook, and you should notice continued improvement.

A Few More Thoughts

Many times our first thoughts in finding a solution to our pain or sleeplessness is to go to the drugstore to "find pills" which will alleviate the symptoms. For many, that solution may work, although, I have found with Kelly and myself, those solutions haven't been as effective as many of the remedies we can find in our own gardens or in health food stores. In the reference section I have outlined many of the remedies we have found to be helpful. It was always important for me to remember that the way to permanently alleviate the problem was to get rid of the underlying cause. Otherwise we are just putting a "bandage" on the symptoms.

My goal from the beginning was and is to change what I need to change within my lifestyle to create a healthy body. In doing that, the symptoms automatically take care of themselves. This is also a life long maintenance program, which is an important thing to remember. If we go back to our old habits once we feel better, the symptoms may recur as our bodies begin to once again to struggle with remaining healthy.

I chose a more natural means to control our symptoms since we found that if pills helped one problem, they also seemed to create another. For Kelly and myself, I feel the natural forms of sleep enhancers and pain control are much more effective. Experiment on your own and take note of what your body is telling you as far as how the remedy is affecting it. If you notice a different, uncomfortable feeling from taking something, chances are you should try something else. This is where quiet time each day comes in. As a person quiets themselves and their mind, a whole new realm of intuitive feelings can come about, along with a new sense of serenity about the FMS.

In the Reference Section, you will find suggestions on simple helps I have found to be beneficial for myself and Kelly. The teas are made by using the same recipe; one to three teaspoons of leave/flowers to one cup boiling water. I let the leaves/flowers infuse in the boiling water from seven to ten minutes. A small amount of honey can be added to any of the teas, although I have found the flavor of each is very good without sweeteners.

Another herbal sweetener which is considered to be healthier for our systems to digest is a product called "stevia." Check with your local health food store for this product, and use it whenever you need a sweetener for baking or other foods.

The second portion of the Reference Section describes other tools we use to relieve symptoms. As you are working through the front of the day to day section, use this section of the book to reference treatments for symptom relief.

Using and Completing the Workbook

1. Before beginning the daily pages of the workbook, fill out the Health Evaluation Form (HEF) on page 11. Use the numbers from 1-10, with 1 being the least and 10 being the greatest frequency/intensity.
2. Fill in the spaces of the HEF to indicate how you have been feeling in general over the past few days. Each month there will be a HEF form in the workbook to complete. This

will serve as a guide to the improvements you are experiencing as each month continues. Remember, the first 90 days lay the ground work for improvement. And improvement is especially slow in the first 60 days.

3. Beginning with day one, read through all the questions before putting down any answers. Then go back through and take note of changes in diet, exercise, etc. that are to be made during that day.

4. As you complete each task, mark the space behind that task with the proper answer.

5. At the end of the day, rate yourself on a scale of 1-10 as to how you felt during the day.

6. Keep a journal describing what you did during the day, and how you felt before, during and after each task. Record any depressed, happy or general feelings about your mood. This is your journal to write about anything you feel. (Many times as we start feeling better, the changes in our general health may be so gradual that we might not notice them. A daily journal is important because it allows us to recognize the subtle changes that have taken place.)

7. Refer to the Reference section in the back of the book when doing the stretching exercises, or for suggestions regarding pain control and sleep.

You are now ready to begin your journey to better health. Remember, this may take some time. It took me almost a full year to feel well again. I didn't see much improvement before three months, and after that the changes were still very gradual. You could take less or more time depending on your own body and how fast it is able to heal itself.

Many times when I was feeling very bad due to the fibromyalgia, it was difficult for me to comprehend the words I was trying to read. To make the instructions easier to follow, in much of the workbook, I have written numbers using digits rather than words. I hope this will make the workbook easier for you to read also.

DAY 2

Today is a wonderful day! It won't be long and you will start to feel the positive effects of the work you have embarked on. Enjoy knowing you are in the healing process.

If it was difficult to eliminate the foods yesterday, start again today. There is no hurry, but persistence will help you achieve your goal of feeling better.

CHOCOLATE: Allow only 1 serving today. Number of servings today: _____

CARBONATED BEVERAGES: Allow no more than on Day 1. Total number of cans bottles consumed today: _____

COFFEE: Allow no more than total cups consumed on Day 1. Number of cups consumed today: _____

ALCOHOL: Allow no more than total cans/drinks than on Day 1. Write number consumed today: _____

CIGARETTES: Allow no more than total cigarettes on Day 1. Write number smoked today: _____

REFINED SUGARS: Allow no more sweets than one time today. Check this box if sweets were kept to 1 serving today: _____

Today, we will begin to change our eating habits. Red meats are very hard for our bodies to digest. Starting today, for the next 2 weeks try to limit red meats to three or fewer servings per week. Be sure to replace meat protein with one of the following protein-rich foods. Check the box of each protein substitute you have eaten to replace the red meat.

beans	___	tofu	___	eggs	___	sprouts	___
almonds	___	TVP*	___	cashews	___	chicken	___
turkey	___	lobster	___	salmon	___	tuna	___

*TVP is a dehydrated soy product that reconstitutes into a ground beef replacement.

Starting today, drink 8 8-ounce glasses of water. Make a mark on the line to represent each glass consumed so you will be sure to consume a full 8 glasses.

EXERCISE: Walk a total of 10 minutes without stopping. Check here after you walk. _____

STRETCHING EXERCISE: Do exercise plan #2 in "Reference Section" of the book. Check here when finished. _____

SLEEP: Repeat sleep preparation from Day 1.

SUPPLEMENTS: Check here after taking your supplements. _____

ON A SCALE OF 1-10, with 1 indicating symptom free and 10 indicating intense pain, rate how you feel today. _____

JOURNAL OF HOW I FELT TODAY AND WHAT I ACCOMPLISHED

Don't forget to compliment yourself today. Pick a bouquet of flowers, or take a few minutes to read a book. Do something nice for yourself today.

DAY 3

I found it helpful when trying to eliminate chocolate from my diet to keep chocolate bits in the freezer. I could then keep track of how many I ate each day, eating 1 less each day until I could eliminate all chocolate. (I was such a chocoholic, it took 4 months to get it completely out of my diet!)

CHOCOLATE: Allow only 1 serving today. Check here if you had 1 serving. _____

CARBONATED BEVERAGES: Allow no more than on Day 1. Check here only if you kept your consumption down by 2 cans. _____

COFFEE: Allow no more than total cups consumed on Day 1. Number of cups consumed today. _____

ALCOHOL: Allow no more than total on Day 1. Write number consumed today: _____

CIGARETTES: Allow no more than total cigarettes on Day 1. Write number smoked today: _____

REFINED SUGARS: Allow sweets 2 times today. Check here if sweets were kept to 2 servings today: _____

Replace red meat with the following items. Check which item you picked.

beans	_____	tofu	_____	eggs	_____	sprouts	_____
almonds	_____	TVP	_____	cashews	_____	chicken	_____
turkey	_____	lobster	_____	salmon	_____	tuna	_____

EXERCISE: Walk a total of 10 minutes without stopping. Check here after you walk. _____

STRETCHING EXERCISE: Do exercise plan #3. Check here when finished. _____

SLEEP: Repeat sleep preparation from Day 1, or choose another preparation from back of work book.

SUPPLEMENTS: Check here after taking your supplements. _____

ON A SCALE OF 1-10, with 1 being the least intensity of discomfort and 10 being the greatest amount of discomfort, how do you feel today? _____

JOURNAL OF HOW I FELT TODAY AND WHAT I ACCOMPLISHED

Remember, you didn't get this illness overnight. It may take 2-3 months before you are able to notice any difference in how you feel, although you should notice subtle differences before that time. This is quite a demanding journey you have embarked upon. Write a thank-you note from your future self for enduring today's struggle.

DAY 4

You've made it through 3 days—you're doing well. Doesn't it feel good to know you are actually doing something to begin to feel better? You have finally made the choice to begin taking control of your fibromyalgia instead of it controlling you! Give yourself a pat on the back. You can do it—I know you can!

CHOCOLATE: Allow only 1 serving today. Check here if you had 1 serving.   ——

CARBONATED BEVERAGES: Same as Day 3. Check here only if you kept your consumption down by 2 cans.   ——

COFFEE: Allow no more than total cups consumed on Day 1. Number of cups consumed today.   ——

ALCOHOL: Allow no more than total on Day 1. Write number consumed today.   ——

CIGARETTES: Allow no more than total cigarettes on Day 1. Write number smoked today.   ——

REFINED SUGARS: Allow sweets 1 time today. Check here if sweets were kept to 1 serving today.   ——

As with yesterday, try to keep your red meat consumption down. We need less protein than we are generally accustomed to eating. Check the item you picked.

beans	——	tofu	——	eggs	——	sprouts	——
almonds	——	TVP*	——	cashews	——	chicken	——
turkey	——	lobster	——	salmon	——	tuna	——

*TVP is a dehydrated soy product that reconstitutes into a ground beef replacement.

EXERCISE: Walk a total of 10 minutes without stopping. Check here after you walk.   ——

STRETCHING EXERCISE: Do exercise plan #2. Check here when finished.   ——

SLEEP: Repeat sleep preparation from Day 1.

SUPPLEMENTS: Check here after taking your supplements.   ——

ON A SCALE OF 1-10, with 1 indicating symptom free and 10 indicating intense pain, rate how you feel today.   ——

JOURNAL OF HOW I FELT TODAY AND WHAT I ACCOMPLISHED

Remember, you didn't get this illness overnight. It may take 2-3 months before you are able to notice any differences in how you feel, although you should notice subtle differences before that time.

DAY 5

Each day thank your body for working with you in this healing process. This serves two purposes: first, it helps you think about getting better, not just coping, and second, it helps you start thinking healthy instead of thinking about how horrible you feel.

CHOCOLATE: Allow only 1 serving today. Check here if you had 1 serving.   ___

CARBONATED BEVERAGES: Same as Day 1. Check here only if you kept your
consumption down by 2 cans.   ___

COFFEE: Allow no more than total cups consumed on Day 1. Number of cups
consumed today.   ___

ALCOHOL: Allow yourself no more than 3 beers today. Write number consumed today.   ___

CIGARETTES: Allow no more than on Day 1. Write number smoked today.   ___

REFINED SUGARS: Allow sweets 2 times today. Check here if sweets
were kept to 2 servings today.   ___

WATER: Drink 8 glasses of water. Note number of glasses consumed today.   ___

Reduce servings of red meat, or substitute with one of the following.

beans	___	tofu	___	eggs	___	sprouts	___
almonds	___	TVP	___	cashews	___	chicken	___
turkey	___	lobster	___	salmon	___	tuna	___

EXERCISE: Walk a total of 10 minutes without stopping. Check here when finished.   ___

STRETCHING EXERCISE: Do exercise plan #1. Check here when finished.   ___

SLEEP: Repeat sleep preparation from Day 1 or use another from back of workbook.

SUPPLEMENTS: Check here after taking your supplements.   ___

ON A SCALE OF 1-10, with 1 being the least intensity of discomfort and 10 being the greatest amount of discomfort, how do you feel today?   ___

JOURNAL OF HOW I FELT TODAY AND WHAT I ACCOMPLISHED

Before writing in your journal today, sit quietly and allow no thoughts to come to mind except one pleasant picture you have chosen to be there. Sit quietly for approximately 10 minutes. When finished, go ahead and write in your journal.

DAY 6

For back and shoulder pain, use some of the acupressure points in the back of the workbook. Many days I would do the stretching exercises more than 1 time.

CHOCOLATE: Allow only 1 serving today. Check here if you had 1 serving. ___

CARBONATED BEVERAGES: Same as Day 3. Check here only if you kept your consumption down by 2 cans. ___

COFFEE: Allow no more than total on Day 1. Number of cups consumed today. ___

ALCOHOL: Allow no more than on Day 1. Write number consumed today. ___

CIGARETTES: Allow no more than on Day 1. Write number smoked today. ___

REFINED SUGARS: Allow sweets 1 time today. Check here if sweets were kept to 1 serving today. ___

WATER: Drink 8 glasses of water. Note number of glasses consumed today. ___

Reduce servings of red meat, or substitute with one of the following.

beans	___	tofu	___	eggs	___	sprouts	___
almonds	___	TVP*	___	cashews	___	chicken	___
turkey	___	lobster	___	salmon	___	tuna	___

*TVP is a dehydrated soy product that reconstitutes into a ground beef replacement.

EXERCISE: Walk a total of 10 minutes without stopping. Check here when finished. ___

STRETCHING EXERCISE: Do exercise plan #1. Check here when finished. ___

SLEEP: Repeat sleep preparation from Day 1 or use another from back of workbook.

SUPPLEMENTS: Check here after taking your supplements. ___

ON A SCALE OF 1-10, with 1 indicating symptom free and 10 indicating intense pain, rate how you feel today. ___

JOURNAL OF HOW I FELT TODAY AND WHAT I ACCOMPLISHED

Remember, you didn't get this illness overnight. It may take 2-3 months before you are able to notice any differences in how you feel, although you should notice subtle differences before that time.

DAY 7

Take note of your posture. Be sure to stand and sit tall. Any time you can, take deep breaths counting to seven as you inhale, filling your abdomen first, then fill your chest. Hold the breath for a count of five, then let it out to the count of seven.

CHOCOLATE: Allow only 1 serving today. Check here if you had 1 serving. ___

CARBONATED BEVERAGES: Same as Day 1. Check here only if you kept your consumption down by 2 cans. ___

COFFEE: Allow no more total on Day 1. Number of cups consumed today. ___

ALCOHOL: Allow no more than on Day 1. Number consumed today. ___

CIGARETTES: Allow no more than on Day 1. Write number smoked today. ___

REFINED SUGARS: Allow 2 servings of sweets. Check here if sweets were kept to 2 servings today. ___

WATER: Drink 8 glasses of water. Note number of glasses consumed today. ___

Reduce servings of red meat, or substitute with one of the following.

beans	___	tofu	___	eggs	___	sprouts	___
almonds	___	TVP	___	cashews	___	chicken	___
turkey	___	lobster	___	salmon	___	tuna	___

EXERCISE: Walk a total of 10 minutes without stopping. Check here when finished. ___

STRETCHING EXERCISE: Do exercise plan #1. Check here when finished. ___

SLEEP: Repeat sleep preparation from Day 1 or use another from back of workbook.

SUPPLEMENTS: Check here after taking your supplements. ___

ON A SCALE OF 1-10, with 1 being the least intensity of discomfort and 10 being the greatest amount of discomfort, how do you feel today? ___

JOURNAL OF HOW I FELT TODAY AND WHAT I ACCOMPLISHED

Deep breathing helps fill the lungs with much needed oxygen.

DAY 8

You have made it through your first week! Congratulations! Keep up the good work.

CHOCOLATE: Allow only 1 serving today. Check here if you had 1 serving.   ___

CARBONATED BEVERAGES: Same as Day 3. Check here only if you kept your
consumption down by 2 cans.   ___

COFFEE: Allow no more than total on Day 1. Number of cups consumed today.   ___

ALCOHOL: Allow no more than on Day 1. Write number consumed today.   ___

CIGARETTES: Allow no more than on Day 1. Write number smoked today.   ___

REFINED SUGARS: Allow 1 serving of sweets. Check here if sweets
were kept to 1 serving today.   ___

WATER: Drink 8 glasses of water. Note number of glasses consumed today.   ___

As with yesterday, try to keep your red meat consumption down. We need less protein than we are generally accustomed to eating. Check the item you picked.

beans ___	tofu ___	eggs ___	sprouts ___
almonds ___	TVP* ___	cashews ___	chicken ___
turkey ___	lobster ___	salmon ___	tuna ___

*TVP is a dehydrated soy product that reconstitutes into a ground beef replacement.

EXERCISE: Walk a total of 15 minutes without stopping. Check here when finished.   ___

STRETCHING EXERCISE: Do exercise plan #3. Check here when finished.   ___

SLEEP: Repeat sleep preparation from Day 1 or use another from back of workbook.

SUPPLEMENTS: Check here after taking your supplements.   ___

ON A SCALE OF 1-10, with 1 indicating symptom free and 10 indicating intense pain,
rate how you feel today.   ___

JOURNAL OF HOW I FELT TODAY AND WHAT I ACCOMPLISHED

Water consumption is very important to help flush toxins out of our bodies. Think of our bodies as an engine and water is to our bodies as oil is to an engine. If there isn't enough lubrication in an engine, it is soon ruined. Our bodies are much the same, if there isn't enough lubrication (water) it won't run effectively either.

DAY 9

Today take one hour at a time and try to judge nothing during that hour. By judging nothing your mind has a chance to rest and restore itself. This is very important to help the body heal.

CHOCOLATE: Allow only 1 serving today. Check here if you had 1 serving. ___
CARBONATED BEVERAGES: Same as Day 1. Check here only if you kept your consumption down by 2 cans. ___
COFFEE: Allow no more than total on Day 1. Number of cups consumed today. ___
ALCOHOL: Allow no more than on Day 1. Write number consumed today. ___
CIGARETTES: Allow no more than on Day 1. Write number smoked today. ___
REFINED SUGARS: Allow 2 servings of sweets. Check here if sweets were kept to 2 servings today. ___
WATER: Drink 8 glasses of water. Note number of glasses consumed today. ___

Reduce servings of red meat, or substitute with one of the following.

beans	___	tofu	___	eggs	___	sprouts	___
almonds	___	TVP	___	cashews	___	chicken	___
turkey	___	lobster	___	salmon	___	tuna	___

EXERCISE: Walk a total of 10 minutes without stopping. Check here when finished. ___
STRETCHING EXERCISE: Do exercise plan #2. Check here when finished. ___
SLEEP: Repeat sleep preparation from Day 1 or use another from back of workbook.
SUPPLEMENTS: Check here after taking your supplements. ___
ON A SCALE OF 1-10, with 1 being the least intensity of discomfort and 10 being the greatest amount of discomfort, how do you feel today? ___

JOURNAL OF HOW I FELT TODAY AND WHAT I ACCOMPLISHED

It is important to get an appropriate amount of essential fatty acids in our systems each day. A good source of essential fatty acids is flaxseed or flaxseed oil. Essential fatty acids help build the immune system.

DAY 10

Today, as you begin your day, stand up tall, and stretch your arms out to the side, take a deep breath, and thank your body for the healing process taking place within it. Then stretch your arms above your head as far as possible and take another deep breath.

CHOCOLATE: Allow only 1 serving today. Check here if you had 1 serving. ___
CARBONATED BEVERAGES: Drink no more than on Day 1. Check here only if you
kept your consumption down by 2 cans. ___
COFFEE: Allow no more than total on Day 1. Number of cups consumed today. ___
ALCOHOL: Allow no more than on Day 1. Write number consumed today. ___
CIGARETTES: Allow no more than on Day 1. Write number smoked today. ___
REFINED SUGARS: Allow 1 serving of sweets. Check here if sweets
were kept to 1 serving today. ___
WATER: Drink 8 glasses of water. Note number of glasses consumed today. ___

As with yesterday, try to keep your red meat consumption down. We need less protein than we are generally accustomed to eating. Check the item you picked.

beans	___	tofu	___	eggs	___	sprouts	___
almonds	___	TVP	___	cashews	___	chicken	___
turkey	___	lobster	___	salmon	___	tuna	___

EXERCISE: Walk a total of 15 minutes without stopping. Check here when finished. ___
STRETCHING EXERCISE: Do exercise plan #1. Check here when finished. ___
SLEEP: Repeat sleep preparation from Day 1 or use another from back of workbook.
SUPPLEMENTS: Check here after taking your supplements. ___
ON A SCALE OF 1-10, with 1 indicating symptom free and 10 indicating intense pain,
rate how you feel today. ___

JOURNAL OF HOW I FELT TODAY AND WHAT I ACCOMPLISHED

These changes are not easy, and take time to make. Be easy on yourself if you slip during the process of the next 4 months.

DAY 11

It is so important to eat plenty of fresh fruits and vegetables. It is believed our bodies do not metabolize foods in the same manner as a "healthy" body. With that in mind, we need the additional nutritional value from fresh foods than we get from cooked or canned foods.

CHOCOLATE: Allow only 1 serving today. Check here if you had 1 serving. ___

CARBONATED BEVERAGES: Drink no more than on Day 1. Check here only if you kept your consumption down by 2 cans. ___

COFFEE: Allow no more than total on Day 1. Number of cups consumed today. ___

ALCOHOL: Allow no more than on Day 1. Write number consumed today. ___

CIGARETTES: Allow no more than on Day 1. Write number smoked today. ___

REFINED SUGARS: Allow 2 servings of sweets. Check here if sweets were kept to 2 servings today. ___

WATER: Drink 8 glasses of water. Note number of glasses consumed today. ___

Reduce servings of red meat, or substitute with one of the following.

beans	___	tofu	___	eggs	___	sprouts	___
almonds	___	TVP	___	cashews	___	chicken	___
turkey	___	lobster	___	salmon	___	tuna	___

EXERCISE: Walk a total of 10 minutes without stopping. Check here when finished. ___

STRETCHING EXERCISE: Do exercise plan #3. Check here when finished. ___

SLEEP: Repeat sleep preparation from Day 1 or use another from back of workbook.

SUPPLEMENTS: Check here after taking your supplements. ___

ON A SCALE OF 1-10, with 1 being the least intensity of discomfort and 10 being the greatest amount of discomfort, how do you feel today? ___

JOURNAL OF HOW I FELT TODAY AND WHAT I ACCOMPLISHED

Keep trying, these changes get easier the more you do them. They become a way of life. When I eat foods, I shouldn't eat, I don't feel so well, so it has become much easier to keep the eating habits I now use.

DAY 12

If you slip on a day, don't beat yourself up because of it. Know that tomorrow's another day and you can begin again fresh the next day and continue on from this moment.

CHOCOLATE: Allow only 1 serving today. Check here if you had 1 serving. ___
CARBONATED BEVERAGES: Drink no more than on Day 3. Check here only if you kept your consumption the same as Day 3. ___
COFFEE: Allow no more than total on Day 1. Number of cups consumed today. ___
ALCOHOL: Allow no more than on Day 1. Write number consumed today. ___
CIGARETTES: Allow no more than on Day 1. Write number smoked today. ___
REFINED SUGARS: Allow 2 servings of sweets. Check here if sweets were kept to 2 servings today. ___
WATER: Drink 8 glasses of water. Note number of glasses consumed today.

Reduce servings of red meat, or substitute with one of the following.

beans	___	tofu	___	eggs	___	sprouts	___
almonds	___	TVP	___	cashews	___	chicken	___
turkey	___	lobster	___	salmon	___	tuna	___

EXERCISE: Walk a total of 15 minutes without stopping. Check here when finished. ___
STRETCHING EXERCISE: Do exercise plan #2. Check here when finished. ___
SLEEP: Repeat sleep preparation from Day 1 or use another from back of workbook.
SUPPLEMENTS: Check here after taking your supplements. ___
ON A SCALE OF 1-10, with 1 indicating symptom free and 10 indicating intense pain, rate how you feel today. ___

JOURNAL OF HOW I FELT TODAY AND WHAT I ACCOMPLISHED

You are doing great. Keep up the good work!

DAY 13

During the day today, try to think positively about anything you may normally think of being a negative in your life. I always wondered why I had to get FMS, although now after 35 years I can see this is what I needed to go through to be able to help you feel better.

CHOCOLATE: Allow only 1 serving today. Check here if you had 1 serving. ___

CARBONATED BEVERAGES: Drink no more than on Day 1. Check here only if you kept your consumption down by 2 cans. ___

COFFEE: Allow no more than total on Day 1. Number of cups consumed today. ___

ALCOHOL: Allow no more than on Day 1. Write number consumed today. ___

CIGARETTES: Allow no more than on Day 1. Write number smoked today. ___

REFINED SUGARS: Allow 2 servings of sweets. Check here if sweets were kept to 2 servings today. ___

WATER: Drink 8 glasses of water. Note number of glasses consumed today. ___

As with yesterday, try to keep your red meat consumption down. We need less protein than we are generally accustomed to eating. Check the item you picked.

beans	___	tofu	___	eggs	___	sprouts	___
almonds	___	TVP	___	cashews	___	chicken	___
turkey	___	lobster	___	salmon	___	tuna	___

EXERCISE: Walk a total of 10 minutes without stopping. Check here when finished. ___

STRETCHING EXERCISE: Do exercise plan #1. Check here when finished. ___

SLEEP: Repeat sleep preparation from Day 1 or use another from back of workbook.

SUPPLEMENTS: Check here after taking your supplements. ___

ON A SCALE OF 1-10, with 1 being the least intensity of discomfort and 10 being the greatest amount of discomfort, how do you feel today? ___

JOURNAL OF HOW I FELT TODAY AND WHAT I ACCOMPLISHED

You are into the program almost 2 weeks. You are 2 weeks closer to feeling well again!

DAY 14

I have found over the years that once I started embracing life, it started embracing me. What a wonderful feeling!

CHOCOLATE: Allow only 1 serving today. Check here if you had 1 serving. ___

CARBONATED BEVERAGES: Drink no more than on Day 3. Write number of cans consumed today. ___

COFFEE: Allow no more than total on Day 1. Number of cups consumed today. ___

ALCOHOL: Allow no more than on Day 1. Write number consumed today. ___

CIGARETTES: Allow no more than on Day 1. Write number smoked today. ___

REFINED SUGARS: Allow 1 serving of sweets. Check here if sweets were kept to 1 serving today. ___

WATER: Drink 8 glasses of water. Note number of glasses consumed today. ___

As with yesterday, try to keep your red meat consumption down. We need less protein than we are generally accustomed to eating. Check the item you picked.

beans	___	tofu	___	eggs	___	sprouts	___
almonds	___	TVP	___	cashews	___	chicken	___
turkey	___	lobster	___	salmon	___	tuna	___

EXERCISE: Walk a total of 15 minutes without stopping. Check here when finished. ___

STRETCHING EXERCISE: Do exercise plan #1. ___

SLEEP: Repeat sleep preparation from Day 1 or use another from back of workbook.

SUPPLEMENTS: Check here after taking your supplements. ___

ON A SCALE OF 1-10, with 1 indicating symptom free and 10 indicating intense pain, rate how you feel today. ___

JOURNAL OF HOW I FELT TODAY AND WHAT I ACCOMPLISHED

Take some time to enjoy a part of nature. This can be done outdoors at a park, in your own yard or indoors with house plants. You could also watch a nature video or play with a pet.

DAY 15

If FMS is caused from a buildup of toxins, it would be to our benefit to stay away from as many toxic chemicals as possible. Instead of using insecticides to keep ants from coming into your house, try making a strong tea from garlic and spray that around the base of your house.

CHOCOLATE: Allow only 1 serving today. Check here if you had 1 serving. ____

CARBONATED BEVERAGES: Drink no more than on Day 1. Consume 2 less cans than before starting the program. ____

COFFEE: Allow no more than total on Day 1. Number of cups consumed today. ____

ALCOHOL: Allow no more than 3 beers. Write number consumed today. ____

CIGARETTES: Allow no more than on Day 1. Write number smoked today. ____

REFINED SUGARS: Allow 1 serving of sweets. Check here if sweets were kept to 1 serving today. ____

WATER: Drink 8 glasses of water. Note number of glasses consumed today. ____

Reduce servings of red meat, or substitute with one of the following.

beans	___	tofu	___	eggs	___	sprouts	___
almonds	___	TVP	___	cashews	___	chicken	___
turkey	___	lobster	___	salmon	___	tuna	___

EXERCISE: Walk a total of 10 minutes without stopping. Check here when finished. ____

STRETCHING EXERCISE: Do exercise plan #2. Check here when finished. ____

SLEEP: Repeat sleep preparation from Day 1 or use another from back of workbook.

SUPPLEMENTS: Check here after taking your supplements. ____

ON A SCALE OF 1-10, with 1 indicating symptom free and 10 indicating intense pain, rate how you feel today. ____

JOURNAL OF HOW I FELT TODAY AND WHAT I ACCOMPLISHED

Once I stopped using insect sprays in my garden, nature took care of the unwanted insects by allowing the "good" insects to come in and eat the "unwanted" insects.

DAY 16

Can you believe you have already been working on becoming healthy for more than 2 weeks? Concentrate on how good it will feel to do the things you like to do again, and use that to give yourself strength.

CHOCOLATE: Allow only 1 serving today. Check here if you had 1 serving.   ——

CARBONATED BEVERAGES: Drink no more than on Day 3. Consume 2 less cans
than before starting the program.   ——

COFFEE: Allow no more than total on Day 1. Number of cups consumed today.   ——

ALCOHOL: Allow no more than 3 beers. Write number consumed today.   ——

CIGARETTES: Allow no more than on Day 1. Write number smoked today.   ——

REFINED SUGARS: Allow 1 serving of sweets. Check here if sweets
were kept to 1 serving today.   ——

WATER: Drink 8 glasses of water. Note number of glasses consumed today.   ——

Reduce servings of red meat, or substitute with one of the following.

beans	——	tofu	——	eggs	——	sprouts	——
almonds	——	TVP	——	cashews	——	chicken	——
turkey	——	lobster	——	salmon	——	tuna	——

EXERCISE: Walk a total of 15 minutes without stopping. Check here when finished.   ——

STRETCHING EXERCISE: Do exercise plan #2. Check here when finished.   ——

SLEEP: Repeat sleep preparation from Day 1 or use another from back of workbook.

SUPPLEMENTS: Check here after taking your supplements.   ——

ON A SCALE OF 1-10, with 1 indicating symptom free and 10 indicating intense pain,
rate how you feel today.   ——

JOURNAL OF HOW I FELT TODAY AND WHAT I ACCOMPLISHED

I have found that if I don't disturb nature, she takes care of herself.

DAY 17

If you notice a sore throat coming on, gargle with saltwater. A good solution is made with 1 teaspoon salt to 1/4 cup of warm water. Gargle 4 times per day.

CHOCOLATE: Allow only 1 serving today. Check here if you had 1 serving. ___

CARBONATED BEVERAGES: Drink no more than on Day 3. Consume 2 less cans than before starting the program. ___

COFFEE: Allow no more than total on Day 1. Number of cups consumed today. ___

ALCOHOL: Allow no more than 3 beers. Write number consumed today. ___

CIGARETTES: Allow no more than on Day 1. Write number smoked today. ___

REFINED SUGARS: Allow 2 servings of sweets. Check here if sweets were kept to 2 servings today. ___

WATER: Drink 8 glasses of water. Note number of glasses consumed today. ___

Reduce servings of red meat, or substitute with one of the following.

beans	___	tofu	___	eggs	___	sprouts	___
almonds	___	TVP	___	cashews	___	chicken	___
turkey	___	lobster	___	salmon	___	tuna	___

EXERCISE: Walk a total of 10 minutes without stopping. Check here when finished. ___

STRETCHING EXERCISE: Do exercise plan #3. Check here when finished. ___

SLEEP: Repeat sleep preparation from Day 1 or use another from back of workbook.

SUPPLEMENTS: Check here after taking your supplements. ___

ON A SCALE OF 1-10, with 1 being the least intensity of discomfort and 10 being the greatest amount of discomfort, how do you feel today? ___

JOURNAL OF HOW I FELT TODAY AND WHAT I ACCOMPLISHED

Take some time to enjoy nature. This can be done outdoors, at at park or in your own backyard. You could also watch a bird feeder or nature video.

DAY 18

When a virus seems to be coming on, many times it can be headed off by drinking echinacea tea. Echinacea can be obtained from most health food stores.

CHOCOLATE: Allow only 1 serving today. Check here if you had 1 serving. ___
CARBONATED BEVERAGES: Drink 3 fewer cans than on Day 1. Write number of cans consumed today. ___
COFFEE: Drink 1 less cup than on Day 17. Number of cups consumed today. ___
ALCOHOL: Allow no more than on Day 1. Write number consumed today. ___
CIGARETTES: Smoke 2 less than on Day 17. Write number smoked today. ___
REFINED SUGARS: Allow 1 serving of sweets. Check here if sweets were kept to 1 serving today. ___
WATER: Drink 8 glasses of water. Note number of glasses consumed today. ___

Reduce servings of red meat, or substitute with one of the following.

beans	___	tofu	___	eggs	___	sprouts	___
almonds	___	TVP	___	cashews	___	chicken	___
turkey	___	lobster	___	salmon	___	tuna	___

EXERCISE: Walk a total of 15 minutes without stopping. Check here when finished. ___
STRETCHING EXERCISE: Do exercise plan #3. Check here when finished. ___
SLEEP: Repeat sleep preparation from Day 1 or use another from back of workbook.
SUPPLEMENTS: Check here after taking your supplements. ___
ON A SCALE OF 1-10, with 1 indicating symptom free and 10 indicating intense pain, rate how you feel today. ___

JOURNAL OF HOW I FELT TODAY AND WHAT I ACCOMPLISHED

You may find you are very susceptible to viruses. Increasing the consumption of immune helpers such as echinacea may be what your body needs to ward off those nasty bugs.

DAY 19

White flour breaks down in the body in a similar form of white sugar. Try to limit the amount of white breads you eat to one per meal.

CHOCOLATE: Allow only 1 serving today. Check here if you had 1 serving. ___
CARBONATED BEVERAGES: Same as Day 18. Write number of cans consumed. ___
COFFEE: Allow no more than total on Day 18. Number of cups consumed today. ___
ALCOHOL: Allow no more than on Day 18. Write number consumed today. ___
CIGARETTES: Allow no more than on Day 1. Write number smoked today. ___
REFINED SUGARS: Allow 2 servings of sweets. Check here if sweets
were kept to 2 servings today. ___
WATER: Drink 8 glasses of water. Note number of glasses consumed today. ___

Reduce servings of red meat, or substitute with one of the following.

beans	___	tofu	___	eggs	___	sprouts	___
almonds	___	TVP	___	cashews	___	chicken	___
turkey	___	lobster	___	salmon	___	tuna	___

EXERCISE: Walk a total of 10 minutes without stopping. Check here when finished. ___
STRETCHING EXERCISE: Do exercise plan #1. Check here when finished. ___
SLEEP: Repeat sleep preparation from Day 1 or use another from back of workbook.
SUPPLEMENTS: Check here after taking your supplements. ___
ON A SCALE OF 1-10, with 1 being the least intensity of discomfort and 10 being the greatest amount of discomfort, how do you feel today? ___

JOURNAL OF HOW I FELT TODAY AND WHAT I ACCOMPLISHED

Feeling well may take a while, but before long, you should start to notice some slight changes. Keep trying, you'll get there!

DAY 20

Today in your journal entry, write down one goal you would like to achieve when you are feeling better. Hold that goal in your mind, and know you will eventually reach this goal.

CHOCOLATE: Allow only 1 serving today. Check here if you had 1 serving. ____
CARBONATED BEVERAGES: Drink 3 fewer cans than on Day 1. Write number
of cans consumed. ____
COFFEE: Drink one less cup than on Day 17. Number of cups consumed today. ____
ALCOHOL: Allow no more than on Day 1. Write number consumed today. ____
CIGARETTES: Smoke 2 less than on Day 17. Write number smoked today. ____
REFINED SUGARS: Allow 1 serving of sweets. Check here if sweets
were kept to 1 serving today. ____
WATER: Drink 8 glasses of water. Note number of glasses consumed today. ____

As with yesterday, try to keep your red meat consumption down. We need less protein than we are generally accustomed to eating. Check the item you picked.

beans	____	tofu	____	eggs	____	sprouts	____
almonds	____	TVP	____	cashews	____	chicken	____
turkey	____	lobster	____	salmon	____	tuna	____

EXERCISE: Walk a total of 15 minutes without stopping. Check here when finished. ____
STRETCHING EXERCISE: Do exercise plan #1. Check here when finished. ____
SLEEP: Repeat sleep preparation from Day 1 or use another from back of workbook.
SUPPLEMENTS: Check here after taking your supplements. ____
ON A SCALE OF 1-10, with 1 indicating symptom free and 10 indicating intense pain,
rate how you feel today. ____

JOURNAL OF HOW I FELT TODAY AND WHAT I ACCOMPLISHED

Try not to be judgmental of anything or any person for an hour today.

DAY 21

It is not uncommon after having a few good days to fall back into a form of relapse, which many times seems as bad as before you began the program. Continue on the program and you will start to feel better.

CHOCOLATE: Allow only 1 serving today. Check here if you had 1 serving. ___
CARBONATED BEVERAGES: Drink 3 fewer cans than on Day 1. Write number
of cans consumed. ___
COFFEE: Allow no more than total on Day 18. Number of cups consumed today. ___
ALCOHOL: Allow no more than on Day 18. Write number consumed today. ___
CIGARETTES: Allow no more than on Day 17. Write number smoked today. ___
REFINED SUGARS: Allow 2 servings of sweets. Check here if sweets
were kept to 2 servings today. ___
WATER: Drink 8 glasses of water. Note number of glasses consumed today. ___

As with yesterday, try to keep your red meat consumption down. We need less protein than we are generally accustomed to eating. Check the item you picked.

beans	___	tofu	___	eggs	___	sprouts	___
almonds	___	TVP	___	cashews	___	chicken	___
turkey	___	lobster	___	salmon	___	tuna	___

EXERCISE: Walk a total of 10 minutes without stopping. Check here when finished. ___
STRETCHING EXERCISE: Do exercise plan #2. Check here when finished. ___
SLEEP: Continue with ideas from back of workbook.
SUPPLEMENTS: Check here after taking your supplements. ___
ON A SCALE OF 1-10, with 1 being the least intensity of discomfort and 10 being the greatest amount of discomfort, how do you feel today? ___

JOURNAL OF HOW I FELT TODAY AND WHAT I ACCOMPLISHED

At Day 30 we will begin to make more changes in your diet. Be prepared.

DAY 22

Instead of looking for that front parking place, begin parking farther out in the parking lot and walking the extra distance. Remember that it is our goal to eliminate these four foods from our diets in the next 4 months: chocolate, carbonated beverages, coffee, and alcohol. Smoking will also be eliminated, and refined sugars will need to be reduced. We will work on eliminating these foods gradually, so you will be able to work them out of your eating habits. If it works better for you to just "cut them out," then do it. Do what works best for you

CHOCOLATE: Allow only 1 serving today. Check here if you had 1 serving.   —

CARBONATED BEVERAGES: Drink no more than on Day 18. Write number
of cans consumed.   —

COFFEE: Allow no more than total on Day 18. Number of cups consumed today.   —

ALCOHOL: Allow no more than on Day 18. Write number consumed today.   —

CIGARETTES: Allow no more than on Day 18. Write number smoked today.   —

REFINED SUGARS: Allow 1 serving of sweets. Check here if sweets
were kept to 1 serving today.   —

WATER: Drink 8 glasses of water. Note number of glasses consumed today.   —

EXERCISE: Walk a total of 15 minutes without stopping. Check here when finished.   —

STRETCHING EXERCISE: Do exercise plan #2. Check here when finished.   —

SLEEP: About 45 minutes before going to bed, take a warm sage bath. Drink a cup of herbal tea, (refer to back of book for sage bath recipe and herbal recommendations). Read about 20 minutes while sitting in a comfortable chair. Go to bed, lay on your back and do deep breathing 3-5 times immediately followed by acupressure points for sleep. (Refer to back of workbook.)

SUPPLEMENTS: Check here after taking your supplements.   —

ON A SCALE OF 1-10, with 1 being the least intensity of discomfort and 10 being the greatest amount of discomfort, how do you feel today?   —

JOURNAL OF HOW I FELT TODAY AND WHAT I ACCOMPLISHED

Increasing exercise is vital to feeling better. Using the large muscles helps get rid of toxins that have built up in the body.

DAY 23

Believe within your heart, with all your being, that you will be healthy again. Any time there is a doubt in your mind, simply remind yourself you are becoming healthy again.

CHOCOLATE: Allow only 1 serving today. Check here if you had 1 serving.   ___

CARBONATED BEVERAGES: Same as on Day 18. Write number of cans consumed.   ___

COFFEE: Allow no more than total on Day 18. Number of cups consumed today.   ___

ALCOHOL: Allow no more than on Day 18. Write number consumed today.   ___

CIGARETTES: Allow no more than on Day 18. Write number smoked today.   ___

REFINED SUGARS: Allow 2 servings of sweets. Check here if sweets were kept to 2 servings today.   ___

WATER: Drink 8 glasses of water. Note number of glasses consumed today.   ___

Eat smaller portions of red meat, or choose a substitute. Check the item you picked.

beans	___	tofu	___	eggs	___	sprouts	___
almonds	___	TVP	___	cashews	___	chicken	___
turkey	___	lobster	___	salmon	___	tuna	___

EXERCISE: Walk a total of 10 minutes without stopping. Check here when finished.   ___

STRETCHING EXERCISE: Do exercise plan #3. Check here when finished.   ___

SLEEP: Continue with ideas from back of workbook.

SUPPLEMENTS: Check here after taking your supplements.   ___

ON A SCALE OF 1-10, with 1 being the least intensity of discomfort and 10 being the greatest amount of discomfort, how do you feel today?   ___

JOURNAL OF HOW I FELT TODAY AND WHAT I ACCOMPLISHED

Health of an individual is not only within the physical body, it is also within the mind and spirit.

DAY 24

Walking is actually good for pain control. By walking many of the large muscles in the back, legs and arms are used. This movement can help reduce pain throughout the body.

CHOCOLATE: Allow only 1 serving today. Check here if you had 1 serving.   ——

CARBONATED BEVERAGES: Drink 3 fewer cans than on Day 1. Write number
of cans consumed.   ——

COFFEE: Allow no more than total on Day 23. Number of cups consumed today.   ——

ALCOHOL: Allow no more than on Day 23. Write number consumed today.   ——

CIGARETTES: Allow no more than on Day 23. Write number smoked today.   ——

REFINED SUGARS: Allow 1 serving of sweets. Check here if sweets
were kept to 1 serving today.   ——

WATER: Drink 8 glasses of water. Note number of glasses consumed today.   ——

Eat smaller portions of red meat, or choose a substitute. Check the item you picked.

beans	——	tofu	——	eggs	——	sprouts	——
almonds	——	TVP	——	cashews	——	chicken	——
turkey	——	lobster	——	salmon	——	tuna	——

EXERCISE: Walk a total of 15 minutes without stopping. Check here when finished.   ——

STRETCHING: Do exercise plan #3. Check here when finished.   ——

SLEEP: Repeat sleep preparation from Day 1, or continue with ideas from back of workbook.

SUPPLEMENTS: Check here after taking your supplements.   ——

ON A SCALE OF 1-10, with 1 indicating symptom free and 10 indicating intense pain,
rate how you feel today.   ——

JOURNAL OF HOW I FELT TODAY AND WHAT I ACCOMPLISHED

When you are feeling extra fatigued, drink another glass of water and breathe deeply a few times.

DAY 25

Garlic is a natural antibiotic, although caution should be used when taking it since it can also lower blood pressure.

CHOCOLATE: Allow only 1 serving today. Check here if you had 1 serving. ___

CARBONATED BEVERAGES: Drink 3 fewer cans than on Day 1. Write number of cans consumed. ___

COFFEE: Allow 2 fewer cups than total on Day 23. Number of cups consumed today. ___

ALCOHOL: Allow 2 fewer drinks than in first week. Write number consumed today. ___

CIGARETTES: Smoke 1 less cigarette than on Day 23. Write number smoked today. ___

REFINED SUGARS: Allow 1 serving of sweets. Check here if sweets were kept to 1 serving today. ___

WATER: Drink 8 glasses of water. Note number of glasses consumed today. ___

If you ate meat yesterday, try not to eat any today. Be sure to replace the protein with one of the following sources. Check the item you picked.

beans ___	tofu ___	eggs ___	sprouts ___
almonds ___	TVP ___	cashews ___	chicken ___
turkey ___	lobster ___	salmon ___	tuna ___

EXERCISE: Walk a total of 15 minutes without stopping. Check here when finished. ___

STRETCHING: Do exercise plan #2. Check here when finished. ___

SLEEP: Repeat sleep preparation from Day 1, or continue with ideas from back of workbook.

SUPPLEMENTS: Check here after taking your supplements. ___

ON A SCALE OF 1-10, with 1 indicating symptom free and 10 indicating intense pain, rate how you feel today. ___

JOURNAL OF HOW I FELT TODAY AND WHAT I ACCOMPLISHED

You have been doing very well. You are nearing the 30-day mark. Keep working, every day you work will bring you closer to better health.

DAY 26

Echinacea is also a natural antibiotic and immune booster. It is better known as "coneflower" and is a perennial herb.

CHOCOLATE: Allow only 1 serving today. Check here if you had 1 serving. ____

CARBONATED BEVERAGES: Drink 3 fewer cans than on Day 1. Write number of cans consumed. ____

COFFEE: Allow 2 fewer cups than total on Day 23. Number of cups consumed today. ____

ALCOHOL: Allow 2 fewer drinks than in first week. Write number consumed today. ____

CIGARETTES: Smoke 1 less cigarette than on Day 22. Write number smoked today. ____

REFINED SUGARS: Allow 1 serving of sweets. Check here if sweets were kept to 1 serving today. ____

WATER: Drink 8 glasses of water. Note number of glasses consumed today. ____

If you ate meat yesterday, try not to eat any today. Be sure to replace the protein with one of the following sources. Check the item you picked.

beans	____	tofu	____	eggs	____	sprouts	____
almonds	____	TVP	____	cashews	____	chicken	____
turkey	____	lobster	____	salmon	____	tuna	____

EXERCISE: Walk a total of 15 minutes without stopping. Check here when finished. ____

STRETCHING: Do exercise plan #3. Check here when finished. ____

SLEEP: Repeat sleep preparation from Day 1, or continue with ideas from back of workbook.

SUPPLEMENTS: Check here after taking your supplements. ____

ON A SCALE OF 1-10, with 1 indicating symptom free and 10 indicating intense pain, rate how you feel today. ____

JOURNAL OF HOW I FELT TODAY AND WHAT I ACCOMPLISHED

The root of echinacea is the part of the herb that is used. Wait until after the first hard frost in the winter before digging up the root and cleaning it. Chop it up and dry for winter storage.

DAY 27

Approximately 20 percent of Americans are believed to have FMS, although only about 7 percent have been diagnosed as of December 1996.

CHOCOLATE: Allow only 1 serving today. Check here if you had 1 serving. _____

CARBONATED BEVERAGES: Allow 1 less can/bottle than yesterday. Write number of cans consumed. _____

COFFEE: Allow 2 fewer cups than total on Day 23. Number of cups consumed today. _____

ALCOHOL: Allow 2 fewer drinks than in first week. Write number consumed today. _____

CIGARETTES: Smoke 2 fewer cigarettes than on Day 23. Write number smoked today. _____

REFINED SUGARS: Allow 2 servings of sweets. Check here if sweets were kept to 2 servings today. _____

WATER: Drink 8 glasses of water. Note number of glasses consumed today. _____

Though it is important to have protein in our diets, it doesn't need to come from red meat only. Try one of the below listed alternatives. Check the item you picked.

beans	_____	tofu	_____	eggs	_____	sprouts	_____
almonds	_____	TVP	_____	cashews	_____	chicken	_____
turkey	_____	lobster	_____	salmon	_____	tuna	_____

EXERCISE: Walk a total of 20 minutes without stopping. Check here when finished. _____

STRETCHING: Do exercise plan #1. Check here when finished. _____

SLEEP: Repeat sleep preparation from Day 1, or continue with ideas from back of workbook.

SUPPLEMENTS: Check here after taking your supplements. _____

ON A SCALE OF 1-10, with 1 indicating the least intensity, rate how you feel today. _____

JOURNAL OF HOW I FELT TODAY AND WHAT I ACCOMPLISHED

If you know of anyone who seems to have symptoms of FMS, don't hesitate to lend them a concerned ear. We all need support to get better.

DAY 28

Whole wheat breads are more nutritious than white breads because the wheat has not been processed as much as the white flour.

CHOCOLATE: Allow only 1 serving today. Check here if you had 1 serving. ____

CARBONATED BEVERAGES: Allow 1 less can/bottle than yesterday. Write number of cans consumed. ____

COFFEE: Allow 2 fewer cups than total on Day 23. Number of cups consumed today. ____

ALCOHOL: Allow 2 fewer drinks than in the first week. Write number consumed. ____

CIGARETTES: Smoke 2 fewer cigarettes than on Day 23. Write number smoked today. ____

REFINED SUGARS: Allow 2 servings of sweets. Check here if sweets were kept to 2 servings today. ____

WATER: Drink 8 glasses of water. Note number of glasses consumed today. ____

Though it is important to have protein in our diets, it doesn't need to come from red meat only. Try one of the below listed alternatives. Check the item you picked.

beans	____	tofu	____	eggs	____	sprouts	____
almonds	____	TVP	____	cashews	____	chicken	____
turkey	____	lobster	____	salmon	____	tuna	____

EXERCISE: Walk a total of 15 minutes without stopping. Check here when finished. ____

STRETCHING: Do exercise plan #2. Check here when finished. ____

SLEEP: Repeat sleep preparation from Day 1, or continue with ideas from back of workbook.

SUPPLEMENTS: Check here after taking your supplements. ____

ON A SCALE OF 1-10, with 1 indicating the least intensity, rate how you feel today. ____

JOURNAL OF HOW I FELT TODAY AND WHAT I ACCOMPLISHED

There are many other flours that can be used for baking instead of white flours. These include brown rice flour, amaranth flour, oat flour and grain flours. The texture in baked goods will be a little different, but these flours are very healthy and don't break down in the same manner in our systems as white flours do.

DAY 29

You've worked very hard. Do something nice for yourself today.

CHOCOLATE: Allow only 1 serving today. Check here if you had 1 serving.

CARBONATED BEVERAGES: Allow 1 less can/bottle than yesterday. Write number of cans consumed. ___

COFFEE: Allow 2 fewer cups than total on Day 23. Number of cups consumed today. ___

ALCOHOL: Allow 2 fewer drinks than in the first week. Write number consumed. ___

CIGARETTES: Smoke 2 fewer cigarettes than on Day 23. Write number smoked today. ___

REFINED SUGARS: Allow 2 servings of sweets. Check here if sweets were kept to 2 servings today.

WATER: Drink 8 glasses of water. Note number of glasses consumed today. ___

Replace red meat with one of the below listed alternatives. Check the item you picked.

beans	___	tofu	___	eggs	___	sprouts	___
almonds	___	TVP	___	cashews	___	chicken	___
turkey	___	lobster	___	salmon	___	tuna	___

EXERCISE: Walk a total of 20 minutes without stopping. Check here when finished. ___

STRETCHING: Do exercise plan #1. Check here when finished. ___

SLEEP: Repeat sleep preparation from Day 1, or continue with ideas from back of workbook.

SUPPLEMENTS: Check here after taking your supplements. ___

ON A SCALE OF 1-10, with 1 indicating the least intensity, rate how you feel today. ___

JOURNAL OF HOW I FELT TODAY AND WHAT I ACCOMPLISHED

You are almost 1/4 of the way through this program. Before long you should notice some changes in how you feel if you aren't noticing changes already.

DAY 30!

You've created a milestone for yourself. It takes approximately 30 days to change a habit. You are well on your way to creating a healthier, happier life!

CHOCOLATE: Allow only 1 serving today. Check here if you had 1 serving.   ___
CARBONATED BEVERAGES: Allow 1 less can/bottle than yesterday. Write number
of cans consumed.   ___
COFFEE: Allow 2 fewer cups than total on Day 23. Number of cups consumed today.   ___
ALCOHOL: Allow 2 fewer drinks than in the first week. Write number consumed.   ___
CIGARETTES: Smoke 2 fewer cigarettes than on Day 23. Write number smoked today.   ___
REFINED SUGARS: Allow 2 servings of sweets. Check here if sweets were kept to 2
servings today.   ___
WATER: Drink 8 glasses of water. Note number of glasses consumed today.   ___

Try to limit red meat to 1 or 2 times a week. Replace red meat with one of the below listed protein alternatives. Check the item you picked.

beans	___	tofu	___	eggs	___	sprouts	___
almonds	___	TVP	___	cashews	___	chicken	___
turkey	___	lobster	___	salmon	___	tuna	___

EXERCISE: Walk a total of 20 minutes without stopping. Check here when finished.   ___
STRETCHING: Do exercise plan #2. Check here when finished.   ___
SLEEP: Repeat sleep preparation from Day 1, or continue with ideas from back of workbook.
SUPPLEMENTS: Check here after taking your supplements.   ___
ou feel today.   ___

JOURNAL OF HOW I FELT TODAY AND WHAT I ACCOMPLISHED

Congratulations! You've succeeded in changing an old habit. Let's begin working on some new changes.

Health Evaluation Form

Refer back to this page only one time per month; after you have filled out the HEF for the next month.

Indicate in the column next to the symptoms which of the following conditions apply to you in terms of frequency and/or intensity of symptoms using the numbers 1-10: 1 being the least amount of intensity and 10 being the greatest. After filling it out, refer to the HEF form filled out in the front section of the workbook to compare the differences.

Low energy/Often feel tired			Light sleep/aware of surroundings	
Skin problems–dry, itchy, acne			Cold hands and feet	
Headaches/migraines			Shortness of breath	
Aching joints			Often feel bloated	
Muscle cramps			Bowel gas	
Menstrual cramps/moody/PMS				
			Heartburn/indigestion	
Cuts and bruises heal slowly			Constipation/diarrhea	
Poor concentration			Weak fingernails/Unhealthy hair	
Difficulty handling stress				
			Poor muscle tone	
Strong desire for sweets/salts			Water retention	
High/low blood pressure			Cellulite	
Frequently take pain killers				
			Allergies/Hayfever	
Moods of depression			Poor night vision	
Difficulty getting up in morning			Varicose veins	
Difficulty falling asleep			Hemorrhoids	

How many glasses of water do you drink each day? ____

How many cups of coffee do you drink each day? ____

How many times do you drink alcohol each day? ____

How many cans of pop do you drink each day? ____

How many times do you eat chocolate each day? ____

How many times do you eat red meat each day? ____

How much weight have you gained in the past year? ____

Congratulations!

You made it through your first 30 days. Congratulations! By now you should be starting to notice some subtle changes. I suppose it could be likened to being in the first trimester of pregnancy. Keep up the good work! Maybe think of this period as being a phase of pregnancy that you are well into. I realize this thought may be tough for you guys. GOOD WORK!

My Gift to You

I tried to climb the mountain top of prosperity,
But each time came tumbling down, thinking God had forgotten me.
And each time I came tumbling down the pain would get stronger
Until at last, I gave in, and knew I needed longer.
To learn the things nature held in her hand, asking me to try each, and every one until I learned why.
Each time I came tumbling down that mountain top was a lesson,
I was to take out to the world, to help each and every person
who, like me, was having pain.
And give the hope into their hearts
That they too, could feel good again.
So, my friend, my gift to you is to know someone cares
to see you once again climbing the hill to health.
And knowing all the way you will be in my prayers.

Mary Moeller

DAY 31

We will begin working on increasing exercise during this 30 days to help create deeper sleep and diminished pain.

CHOCOLATE: Starting today you will cut chocolate down to 1 serving every other day. Cut amount in your servings to half of day 29. Note the day and amount eaten.   ___

CARBONATED BEVERAGES: Today allow no more than 2 cans of carbonated beverages. Enter amount consumed.   ___

COFFEE: Allow no more than 3 cups today. Number of cups consumed today.   ___

ALCOHOL: Allow no more than 1 drink today. Write number consumed.   ___

CIGARETTES: Smoke 2 fewer cigarettes than on Day 23. Write number smoked today.   ___

REFINED SUGARS: Limit sugars to 1 serving and white bread to 2 servings. Enter number of times consumed.   ___

WATER: Drink 8 glasses of water. Note number of glasses consumed today.   ___

Try to limit red meat to 1 or 2 times a week. Replace red meat with one of the below listed protein alternatives. Check the item you picked.

beans	___	tofu	___	eggs	___	sprouts	___
almonds	___	TVP	___	cashews	___	chicken	___
turkey	___	lobster	___	salmon	___	tuna	___

EXERCISE: Increase time to 25 minutes without stopping. Check here when finished.   ___

STRETCHING: Do exercise plan #3. Check here when finished.   ___

SLEEP: Repeat sleep preparation from Day 1, or continue with ideas from back of workbook.

SUPPLEMENTS: Check here after taking your supplements.   ___

ON A SCALE OF 1-10, with 1 indicating the least intensity, how you feel today?   ___

JOURNAL OF HOW I FELT TODAY AND WHAT I ACCOMPLISHED

Papaya is a very effective aid for upset stomach. It can be purchased in small square pieces and kept in a bag in your pocket or purse.

DAY 32

When drinking coffee, the decaffeinated brands are just as detrimental to our systems as the caffeinated brands.

CHOCOLATE: Keep chocolate down to 1 serving every other day. Cut the amount of your servings to half of day 29. Note the amount eaten. ___

CARBONATED BEVERAGES: Allow no more than 2 cans. Enter amount consumed. ___

COFFEE: Allow no more than 3 cups today. Number of cups consumed today. ___

ALCOHOL: Allow no more than 1 drink today. Write number consumed. ___

CIGARETTES: Try to smoke less than 6 cigarettes (if not there already). Write number smoked today. ___

REFINED SUGARS: Limit sugars to 2 servings today. Enter number of times consumed. ___

WATER: Drink 8 glasses of water. Note number of glasses consumed today. ___

Try to limit red meat to 1 or 2 times a week. Replace red meat with one of the below listed protein alternatives. Check the item you picked.

beans	___	tofu	___	eggs	___	sprouts	___
almonds	___	TVP	___	cashews	___	chicken	___
turkey	___	lobster	___	salmon	___	tuna	___

EXERCISE: Increase time to 25 minutes without stopping. Check here when finished. ___

STRETCHING: Do exercise plan #1. Check here when finished. ___

SLEEP: Repeat sleep preparation from Day 1, or continue with ideas from back of workbook.

SUPPLEMENTS: Check here after taking your supplements. ___

ON A SCALE OF 1-10, with 1 indicating the least intensity, how you feel today? ___

JOURNAL OF HOW I FELT TODAY AND WHAT I ACCOMPLISHED

If you must drink coffee, try the organic kinds. Some doctors feel the chemicals sprayed on the bean while it is growing contributes to FMS symptoms.

DAY 33

A good replacement for carbonated beverages is a glass of ice cold water with lemon in it.

CHOCOLATE: Keep chocolate down to 1 serving every other day. Keep amount in serving the same as Day 32. Note the amount eaten. ___

CARBONATED BEVERAGES: Allow no more than 2 cans. Enter amount consumed. ___

COFFEE: Allow no more than 3 cups today. Number of cups consumed today. ___

ALCOHOL: Allow no more than 3 drinks today. Write number consumed. ___

CIGARETTES: Try to smoke less than 6 cigarettes (if not there already). Write number smoked today. ___

REFINED SUGARS: Limit sugars to 1 serving today. Enter number of times consumed. ___

WATER: Drink 8 glasses of water. Note number of glasses consumed today. ___

Try to limit red meat to 2 servings a week. Replace red meat with one of the below listed protein alternatives. Check the item you picked.

beans	___	tofu	___	eggs	___	sprouts	___
almonds	___	TVP	___	cashews	___	chicken	___
turkey	___	lobster	___	salmon	___	tuna	___

EXERCISE: Increase time to 25 minutes without stopping. Check here when finished. ___

STRETCHING: Do exercise plan #2. Check here when finished. ___

SLEEP: Repeat sleep preparation from Day 1, or continue with ideas from back of workbook.

SUPPLEMENTS: Check here after taking your supplements. ___

ON A SCALE OF 1-10, with 1 indicating the least intensity, how you feel today? ___

JOURNAL OF HOW I FELT TODAY AND WHAT I ACCOMPLISHED

Lemon juice in cold water eliminates the craving for carbonation. Didn't I just say that?

DAY 34

Flavored yogurt contains artificial sweeteners which are difficult for our bodies to digest. Try adding your own fruits to plain yogurt. Be sure to check that the plain yogurt you choose doesn't have artificial sweeteners in it.

CHOCOLATE: Keep chocolate down to 1 serving every other day. Keep serving amount the same as Day 33. Note the amount eaten. ___

CARBONATED BEVERAGES: Allow no more than 2 cans. Enter amount consumed. ___

COFFEE: Allow no more than 3 cups today. Number of cups consumed today. ___

ALCOHOL: Allow no more than 3 drinks today. Write number consumed. ___

CIGARETTES: Try to smoke less than 6 cigarettes. Write number smoked today. ___

REFINED SUGARS: Limit sugars to 1 serving and white bread to 2 servings today. Enter number of times consumed. ___

WATER: Drink one more glass than on day 33. Note number of glasses consumed. ___

Try to limit red meat to 2 servings a week. Replace red meat with one of the below listed protein alternatives. Check the item you picked.

beans	___	tofu	___	eggs	___	sprouts	___
almonds	___	TVP	___	cashews	___	chicken	___
turkey	___	lobster	___	salmon	___	tuna	___

EXERCISE: Increase time to 25 minutes without stopping. Check here when finished. ___

STRETCHING: Do exercise plan #3. Check here when finished. ___

SLEEP: Repeat sleep preparation from Day 1, or continue with ideas from back of workbook.

SUPPLEMENTS: Check here after taking your supplements. ___

ON A SCALE OF 1-10, with 1 indicating the least intensity, how you feel today? ___

JOURNAL OF HOW I FELT TODAY AND WHAT I ACCOMPLISHED

If possible try to find unsweetened brands of yogurt and add your own sweetener.

DAY 35

If you find you are craving something sweet about mid-morning and mid-afternoon, eat a piece of fruit or drink a small glass of juice or milk.

CHOCOLATE: Keep chocolate down to 1 serving every other day. Keep serving amount the same as Day 33. Note the amount eaten. ___

CARBONATED BEVERAGES: Allow no more than 2 cans. Enter amount consumed. ___

COFFEE: Allow no more than 3 cups today. Number of cups consumed today. ___

ALCOHOL: Allow no more than 3 drinks today. Write number consumed. ___

CIGARETTES: Try to smoke 6 or fewer cigarettes (if not there already). Write number smoked today. ___

REFINED SUGARS: Limit sugars to 1 serving and white bread to 2 servings today. Enter number of servings consumed. ___

WATER: Drink 8 glasses of water. Note number of glasses consumed. ___

Try to limit red meat to 2 servings a week. Replace red meat with one of the below listed protein alternatives. Check the item you picked.

beans ___	tofu ___	eggs ___	sprouts ___
almonds ___	TVP ___	cashews ___	chicken ___
turkey ___	lobster ___	salmon ___	tuna ___

EXERCISE: Increase time to 25 minutes without stopping. Check here when finished. ___

STRETCHING: Do exercise plan #1. Check here when finished. ___

SLEEP: Continue with ideas from back of workbook.

SUPPLEMENTS: Check here after taking your supplements. ___

ON A SCALE OF 1-10, with 1 indicating the least intensity, how you feel today? ___

JOURNAL OF HOW I FELT TODAY AND WHAT I ACCOMPLISHED

A small snack around 2 and 4 o'clock in the afternoon can help with sugar cravings. Keep the snack healthy and small. Drink another small glass of juice or have some fruit again before going to bed.

DAY 36

Try using bananas on your cereal instead of sugar. Strawberries or other sweet fruit are good replacements for sugar.

CHOCOLATE: Keep chocolate down to 1 serving every other day. Keep amount of serving to half of Day 29. Note the amount eaten. ___

CARBONATED BEVERAGES: Allow no more than 2 cans. Enter amount consumed. ___

COFFEE: Allow no more than 3 cups today. Number of cups consumed today. ___

ALCOHOL: Allow no more than 3 drinks today. Write number consumed. ___

CIGARETTES: Try to smoke 6 or fewer cigarettes. Write number smoked today. ___

REFINED SUGARS: Limit sugars to 1 serving and white bread to 2 servings today. Enter number of servings consumed. ___

WATER: Drink 8 glasses of water. Note number of glasses consumed. ___

Try to limit red meat to 2 servings a week. Replace red meat with one of the below listed protein alternatives. Check the item you picked.

beans	___	tofu	___	eggs	___	sprouts	___
almonds	___	TVP	___	cashews	___	chicken	___
turkey	___	lobster	___	salmon	___	tuna	___

EXERCISE: Increase time to 25 minutes without stopping. Check here when finished. ___

STRETCHING: Do exercise plan #2. Check here when finished. ___

SLEEP: Continue with ideas from back of workbook.

SUPPLEMENTS: Check here after taking your supplements. ___

ON A SCALE OF 1-10, with 1 indicating the least intensity, how you feel today? ___

JOURNAL OF HOW I FELT TODAY AND WHAT I ACCOMPLISHED

Try mixing sweet fruits with tart fruits, and if they need sweetening try using either fructose or stevia for sweeteners.

DAY 37

I put rolled oats into my blender and blend until it is the consistency of flour to use for my baking needs.

CHOCOLATE: Keep chocolate down to 1 serving every other day. Keep amount of serving to half of Day 29. Note the amount eaten.   ___
CARBONATED BEVERAGES: Allow no more than 2 cans. Enter amount consumed.   ___
COFFEE: Allow no more than 3 cups today. Number of cups consumed today.   ___
ALCOHOL: Allow no more than 3 drinks today. Write number consumed.   ___
CIGARETTES: Try to smoke 6 or fewer cigarettes. Write number smoked today.   ___
REFINED SUGARS: Limit sugars to 1 serving and white bread to 2 servings today. Enter number of servings consumed.
WATER: Drink 1 more glasses of water than on Day 23. Note number consumed.   ___

Take note as to how you feel after eating red meat.. Replace red meat with one of the below listed protein alternatives. Check the item you picked.

beans	___	tofu	___	eggs	___	sprouts	___
almonds	___	TVP	___	cashews	___	chicken	___
turkey	___	lobster	___	salmon	___	tuna	___

EXERCISE: Increase time to 25 minutes without stopping. Check here when finished.   ___
STRETCHING: Do exercise plan #3. Check here when finished.   ___
SLEEP: Continue with ideas from back of workbook.
SUPPLEMENTS: Check here after taking your supplements.   ___
ON A SCALE OF 1-10, with 1 indicating the least intensity, how you feel today?   ___

JOURNAL OF HOW I FELT TODAY AND WHAT I ACCOMPLISHED

Use rolled oats blended in blender until consistency of flour for your baking needs. Oat flour can be purchased in many health food stores. Baked goods made with oat flour will tend to be heavier in consistency.

DAY 38

Flour tortilla shells make great low-fat pie crusts! Just put them in the pie pan before the fruit.

CHOCOLATE: Keep chocolate down to 1 serving every other day. Cut amount in your servings to half of regular servings.. Note the amount eaten. ___

CARBONATED BEVERAGES: Allow no more than 2 cans. Enter amount consumed. ___

COFFEE: Allow no more than 3 cups today. Number of cups consumed today. ___

ALCOHOL: Allow no more than 3 drinks today. Write number consumed. ___

CIGARETTES: Try to smoke 6 or fewer cigarettes. Write number smoked today. ___

REFINED SUGARS: Limit sugars to 1 serving and white bread to 2 servings today. Enter number of servings consumed. ___

WATER: Drink 8 glasses of water. Note number of glasses. ___

Take note as to how you feel after eating red meat.. Replace red meat with one of the below listed protein alternatives. Check the item you picked.

beans	___	tofu	___	eggs	___	sprouts	___
almonds	___	TVP	___	cashews	___	chicken	___
turkey	___	lobster	___	salmon	___	tuna	___

EXERCISE: Increase time to 25 minutes without stopping. Check here when finished. ___

STRETCHING: Do exercise plan #2. Check here when finished. ___

SLEEP: Continue with ideas from back of workbook.

SUPPLEMENTS: Check here after taking your supplements. ___

ON A SCALE OF 1-10, with 1 indicating the least intensity, how you feel today? ___

JOURNAL OF HOW I FELT TODAY AND WHAT I ACCOMPLISHED

Use tapioca for thickening of fruit pies instead of white flour.

DAY 39

When making burritos, try using beans (red, white, navy, or any kind) in place of meat. Delicious, nutritious and low in fat!

CHOCOLATE: Keep chocolate down to 1 serving every other day. Cut amount in your servings to half of regular servings. Note the amount eaten. ___

CARBONATED BEVERAGES: Allow no more than 2 cans. Enter amount consumed. ___

COFFEE: Allow no more than 3 cups today. Number of cups consumed today. ___

ALCOHOL: Allow no more than 3 drinks today. Write number consumed. ___

CIGARETTES: Try to smoke 6 or fewer cigarettes. Write number smoked today. ___

REFINED SUGARS: Limit sugars to 1 serving and white bread to 2 servings today. Enter number of servings consumed. ___

WATER: Drink 8 glasses of water. Note number of glasses. ___

Take note as to how you feel after eating red meat.. Replace red meat with one of the below listed protein alternatives. Check the item you picked.

beans	___	tofu	___	eggs	___	sprouts	___
almonds	___	TVP	___	cashews	___	chicken	___
turkey	___	lobster	___	salmon	___	tuna	___

EXERCISE: Increase time to 25 minutes without stopping. Check here when finished. ___

STRETCHING: Do exercise plan #3. Check here when finished. ___

SLEEP: Continue with ideas from back of workbook.

SUPPLEMENTS: Check here after taking your supplements. ___

ON A SCALE OF 1-10, with 1 indicating the least intensity, how you feel today? ___

JOURNAL OF HOW I FELT TODAY AND WHAT I ACCOMPLISHED

Mix a little chili powder and paprika into beans before serving for extra Mexican flavor.

DAY 40

Flaxseed is very inexpensive and full of both essential fatty acids and fiber. I add flax seed to my cereals, milk shakes and breakfast drinks.

CHOCOLATE: Keep chocolate down to 1 serving every other day. Cut amount in your servings to half of regular servings.. Note the amount eaten. ___

CARBONATED BEVERAGES: Allow no more than 2 cans. Enter amount consumed. ___

COFFEE: Allow no more than 3 cups today. Number of cups consumed today. ___

ALCOHOL: Allow no more than 3 drinks today. Write number consumed. ___

CIGARETTES: Try to smoke 6 or fewer cigarettes. Write number smoked today. ___

REFINED SUGARS: Limit sugars to 1 serving and white bread to 2 servings today. Enter number of servings consumed. ___

WATER: Drink 8 glasses of water. Note number of glasses. ___

Take note as to how you feel after eating red meat.. Replace red meat with one of the below listed protein alternatives. Check the item you picked.

beans	___	tofu	___	eggs	___	sprouts	___
almonds	___	TVP	___	cashews	___	chicken	___
turkey	___	lobster	___	salmon	___	tuna	___

EXERCISE: Increase time to 25 minutes without stopping. Check here when finished. ___

STRETCHING: Do exercise plan #2. Check here when finished. ___

SLEEP: Continue with ideas from back of workbook.

SUPPLEMENTS: Check here after taking your supplements. ___

ON A SCALE OF 1-10, with 1 indicating the least intensity, how you feel today? ___

JOURNAL OF HOW I FELT TODAY AND WHAT I ACCOMPLISHED

Adding 1 to 2 tablespoons flaxseed to your diet each day can help reduce pain and constipation.

DAY 41

Many people have noticed reduced pain after taking flaxseed over a period of a few weeks.

CHOCOLATE: Continue to cut chocolate down to 1 serving every other day. Cut amount in your servings to half of regular servings.. Note the amount eaten.   ___
CARBONATED BEVERAGES: Allow no more than 2 cans. Enter amount consumed.   ___
COFFEE: Allow no more than 3 cups today. Number of cups consumed today.   ___
ALCOHOL: Allow no more than 3 drinks today. Write number consumed.   ___
CIGARETTES: Try to smoke 6 or fewer cigarettes. Write number smoked today.   ___
REFINED SUGARS: Limit sugars to 1 serving and white bread to 2 servings today. Enter number of servings consumed.   ___
WATER: Drink 9 glasses of water. Note number of glasses.   ___

You can eat red meat 2 times per week now. Notice how you feel after eating it. Replace red meat with one of the listed protein alternatives. Check the item you picked.

beans	___	tofu	___	eggs	___	sprouts	___
almonds	___	TVP	___	cashews	___	chicken	___
turkey	___	lobster	___	salmon	___	tuna	___

EXERCISE: Increase time to 25 minutes without stopping. Check here when finished.   ___
STRETCHING: Do exercise plan #1. Check here when finished.   ___
SLEEP: Continue with ideas from back of workbook.
SUPPLEMENTS: Check here after taking your supplements.   ___
ON A SCALE OF 1-10, with 1 indicating the least intensity, how you feel today?   ___

JOURNAL OF HOW I FELT TODAY AND WHAT I ACCOMPLISHED

Flaxseed contains essential fats necessary for our bodies to function properly. The typical American is low on this form of fat.

DAY 42

To make my life easier, and to keep cooking down to a minimum, I try to make double of the servings of food my family will eat in a typical meal. Then I freeze the rest of the meal for another time.

CHOCOLATE: Continue to cut chocolate down to 1 serving every other day. Cut amount in your servings to half of regular servings.. Note the amount eaten. ___

CARBONATED BEVERAGES: Allow no more than 2 cans. Enter amount consumed. ___

COFFEE: Allow no more than 3 cups today. Number of cups consumed today. ___

ALCOHOL: Allow no more than 3 drinks today. Write number consumed. ___

CIGARETTES: Try to smoke 6 or fewer cigarettes. Write number smoked today. ___

REFINED SUGARS: Limit sugars to 1 serving and white bread to 2 servings today. Enter number of servings consumed. ___

WATER: Drink 8 glasses of water. Note number of glasses. ___

You can eat red meat 2 times per week now. Notice how you feel after eating it. Replace red meat with one of the listed protein alternatives. Check the item you picked.

beans	___	tofu	___	eggs	___	sprouts	___
almonds	___	TVP	___	cashews	___	chicken	___
turkey	___	lobster	___	salmon	___	tuna	

EXERCISE: Increase time to 25 minutes without stopping. Check here when finished. ___

STRETCHING: Do exercise plan #2. Check here when finished. ___

SLEEP: Continue with ideas from back of workbook.

SUPPLEMENTS: Check here after taking your supplements. ___

ON A SCALE OF 1-10, with 1 indicating the least intensity, how you feel today? ___

JOURNAL OF HOW I FELT TODAY AND WHAT I ACCOMPLISHED

Left over plastic dinner plates from frozen entrees such as "TV dinners" can be used again by adding leftovers from dinner to create a new frozen dinner. It's nice to have them on those nights you don't feel like cooking.

DAY 43

Parsley is very easy to grow and requires little care. One handful of parsley per day can provide many essential nutrients and is a good source of calcium.

CHOCOLATE: Continue to cut chocolate down to 1 serving every other day. Cut amount in your servings to half of regular servings. Note the amount eaten. ___

CARBONATED BEVERAGES: Allow no more than 1 can. Enter amount consumed. ___

COFFEE: Allow no more than 3 cups today. Number of cups consumed today. ___

ALCOHOL: Allow no more than 3 drinks today. Write number consumed. ___

CIGARETTES: Try to smoke 6 or fewer cigarettes. Write number smoked today. ___

REFINED SUGARS: Limit sugars to 1 serving and white bread to 2 servings today. Enter number of servings consumed. ___

WATER: Drink 8 glasses of water. Note number of glasses. ___

When I didn't feel well after eating red meat, I cut it out of my diet for 2 weeks, and replace it with one of the following. Check the item you picked.

beans	___	tofu	___	eggs	___	sprouts	___
almonds	___	TVP	___	cashews	___	chicken	___
turkey	___	lobster	___	salmon	___	tuna	___

EXERCISE: Increase time to 25 minutes without stopping. Check here when finished. ___

STRETCHING: Do exercise plan #3. Check here when finished. ___

SLEEP: Continue with ideas from back of workbook.

SUPPLEMENTS: Check here after taking your supplements. ___

ON A SCALE OF 1-10, with 1 indicating the least intensity, how you feel today? ___

JOURNAL OF HOW I FELT TODAY AND WHAT I ACCOMPLISHED

To dry parsley, pick around noon on a full moon day and hang upside down in a paper bag. Place bag in a dark room or closet until parsley has dried.

DAY 44

Sage is another perennial herb which requires little care, yet it has so many wonderful uses. Dry as described for parsley.

CHOCOLATE: Continue to cut chocolate down to 1 serving every other day. Cut amount in your servings to half of regular servings. Note the amount eaten. ____

CARBONATED BEVERAGES: Allow no more than 1 can. Enter amount consumed. ____

COFFEE: Allow no more than 3 cups today. Number of cups consumed today. ____

ALCOHOL: Allow no more than 3 drinks today. Write number consumed. ____

CIGARETTES: Try to smoke 6 or fewer cigarettes. Write number smoked today. ____

REFINED SUGARS: Limit sugars to 1 serving and white bread to 2 servings today. Enter number of servings consumed. ____

WATER: Drink 8 glasses of water. Note number of glasses. ____

Note how red meat makes you feel. Check the item you picked.

beans	___	tofu	___	eggs	___	sprouts	___
almonds	___	TVP	___	cashews	___	chicken	___
turkey	___	lobster	___	salmon	___	tuna	___

EXERCISE: Increase time to 30 minutes without stopping. Check here when finished. ____

STRETCHING: Do exercise plan #1. Check here when finished. ____

SLEEP: Continue with ideas from back of workbook.

SUPPLEMENTS: Check here after taking your supplements. ____

ON A SCALE OF 1-10, with 1 indicating the least intensity, how you feel today? ____

JOURNAL OF HOW I FELT TODAY AND WHAT I ACCOMPLISHED

In the summer and fall I hang herbs to dry in my closets to help freshen the air. In the winter it is easy to slide the leaves off for storage in canning jars.

DAY 45

Mint is wonderful for an upset stomach.

CHOCOLATE: Continue to cut chocolate down to 1 serving every other day. Cut amount in your servings to half of regular servings. Note the amount eaten. ___

CARBONATED BEVERAGES: Allow no more than 2 cans. Enter amount consumed. ___

COFFEE: Allow no more than 3 cups today. Number of cups consumed today. ___

ALCOHOL: Allow no more than 3 drinks today. Write number consumed. ___

CIGARETTES: Try to smoke 6 or fewer cigarettes. Write number smoked today. ___

REFINED SUGARS: Limit sugars to 1 serving and white bread to 2 servings today. Enter number of servings consumed.

WATER: Drink 8 glasses of water. Note number of glasses. ___

Replace red meat with one of the following items. Check the item you picked.

beans	___	tofu	___	eggs	___	sprouts	___
almonds	___	TVP	___	cashews	___	chicken	___
turkey	___	lobster	___	salmon	___	tuna	___

EXERCISE: Increase time to 25 minutes without stopping. Check here when finished. ___

STRETCHING: Do exercise plan #2. Check here when finished. ___

SLEEP: Continue with ideas from back of workbook.

SUPPLEMENTS: Check here after taking your supplements. ___

ON A SCALE OF 1-10, with 1 indicating the least intensity, how you feel today? ___

JOURNAL OF HOW I FELT TODAY AND WHAT I ACCOMPLISHED

When my children get the stomach flu, a cup of mint tea will many times settle their stomachs. They usually enjoy relief for more than 3 hours.

DAY 46

Mint has many uses, but should be planted where it has plenty of room to spread. Mint tea many times will settle an upset stomach.

CHOCOLATE: Allow 1 small serving every other day. Note the amount eaten. ____

CARBONATED BEVERAGES: Allow no more than 1 can. Enter amount consumed. ____

COFFEE: Allow no more than 3 cups today. Number of cups consumed today. ____

ALCOHOL: Allow no more than 2 drinks today. Write number consumed. ____

CIGARETTES: Try to smoke 5 or less cigarettes. Write number smoked today. ____

REFINED SUGARS: Limit sugars to 1 serving and white bread to 2 servings today. Enter number of servings consumed. ____

WATER: Drink 8 glasses of water. Note number of glasses. ____

Replace red meat with one of the following items. Check the item you picked.

beans	____	tofu	____	eggs	____	sprouts	____
almonds	____	TVP	____	cashews	____	chicken	____
turkey	____	lobster	____	salmon	____	tuna	____

EXERCISE: Walk briskly for 30 minutes without stopping. Check here when finished. ____

STRETCHING: Do exercise plan #3. Check here when finished. ____

SLEEP: Continue with ideas from back of workbook.

SUPPLEMENTS: Check here after taking your supplements. ____

ON A SCALE OF 1-10, with 1 indicating the least intensity, how you feel today? ____

JOURNAL OF HOW I FELT TODAY AND WHAT I ACCOMPLISHED

Mint also makes a pretty ice mold if placed into water before it is frozen.

DAY 47

A strong peppermint tea can help ward off a cold when taken as soon as symptoms appear.

CHOCOLATE: Allow 1 small serving every other day. Note the amount eaten.   ___

CARBONATED BEVERAGES: Allow no more than 1 can. Enter amount consumed.   ___

COFFEE: Allow no more than 3 cups today. Number of cups consumed today.   ___

ALCOHOL: Allow no more than 3 drinks today. Write number consumed.   ___

CIGARETTES: Try to smoke 5 or less cigarettes. Write number smoked today.   ___

REFINED SUGARS: Limit sugars to 1 serving and white bread to 2 servings today. Enter number of servings consumed.   ___

WATER: Drink 8 glasses of water. Note number of glasses.   ___

Replace red meat with one of the following items. Check the item you picked.

beans	___	tofu	___	eggs	___	sprouts	___
almonds	___	TVP	___	cashews	___	chicken	___
turkey	___	lobster	___	salmon	___	tuna	___

EXERCISE: Walk briskly for 30 minutes without stopping. Check here when finished.   ___

STRETCHING: Do exercise plan #1. Check here when finished.   ___

SLEEP: Continue with ideas from back of workbook.

SUPPLEMENTS: Check here after taking your supplements.   ___

ON A SCALE OF 1-10, with 1 indicating the least intensity, how you feel today?   ___

JOURNAL OF HOW I FELT TODAY AND WHAT I ACCOMPLISHED

Many people with FMS crave salt or salty foods. It has been very beneficial for Kelly and I to watch our consumption of these foods and eliminate them as often as possible. That can be a pretty hard task!

DAY 48

Rubbing mint leaves on the forehead and temples is said to help relieve headaches.

CHOCOLATE: Allow 1 small serving every other day. Keep them in your freezer so you know
they are there to eat. Note the amount eaten.   ____

CARBONATED BEVERAGES: Allow no more than 1 can. Enter amount consumed.   ____

COFFEE: Allow no more than 3 cups today. Number of cups consumed today.   ____

ALCOHOL: Allow no more than 3 drinks today. Write number consumed.   ____

CIGARETTES: Try to smoke 5 or less cigarettes. Write number smoked today.   ____

REFINED SUGARS: Limit sugars to 1 serving and white bread to 2 servings today. Enter
number of servings consumed.   ____

WATER: Drink 8 glasses of water. Note number of glasses.   ____

Replace red meat with one of the following items. Check the item you picked.

beans	____	tofu	____	eggs	____	sprouts	____
almonds	____	TVP	____	cashews	____	chicken	____
turkey	____	lobster	____	salmon	____	tuna	____

EXERCISE: Walk briskly for 30 minutes without stopping. Check here when finished.   ____

STRETCHING: Do exercise plan #1. Check here when finished.   ____

SLEEP: Continue with ideas from back of workbook.

SUPPLEMENTS: Check here after taking your supplements.   ____

ON A SCALE OF 1-10, with 1 indicating the least intensity, how you feel today?   ____

JOURNAL OF HOW I FELT TODAY AND WHAT I ACCOMPLISHED

From here on put the number of glasses of water consumed in each day in the space desig-
nated for water.

DAY 49

Chamomile likes to be placed in an area where it will be stepped on. When mixed with mint and catnip and consumed as a tea, it can be an excellent way to help to get a good night's sleep.

CHOCOLATE: Allow 1 small serving every other day. Keep them in your freezer so you know they are there to eat. Note the amount eaten. ____

CARBONATED BEVERAGES: Allow no more than 1 can. Enter amount consumed. ____

COFFEE: Allow no more than 3 cups today. Number of cups consumed today. ____

ALCOHOL: Allow no more than 3 drinks today. Write number consumed. ____

CIGARETTES: Try to smoke 5 or less cigarettes. Write number smoked today. ____

REFINED SUGARS: Limit sugars to 1 serving and white bread to 2 servings today. Enter number of servings consumed. ____

WATER: Drink 8 glasses of water. Note number of glasses. ____

Replace red meat with one of the following items. Check the item you picked.

beans	____	tofu	____	eggs	____	sprouts	____
almonds	____	TVP	____	cashews	____	chicken	____
turkey	____	lobster	____	salmon	____	tuna	____

EXERCISE: Walk briskly for 30 minutes without stopping. Check here when finished. ____

STRETCHING: Do exercise plan #2. Check here when finished. ____

SLEEP: Continue with ideas from back of workbook.

SUPPLEMENTS: Check here after taking your supplements. ____

ON A SCALE OF 1-10, with 1 indicating the least intensity, how you feel today? ____

JOURNAL OF HOW I FELT TODAY AND WHAT I ACCOMPLISHED

When going out to eat, it has been helpful for us to go to a buffet and eat a plate of fresh vegetables and fruit before going to the hot food bar. We also eat fewer foods that aren't so healthy since we are already partially full.

DAY 50

Catnip is wonderful for relaxation and is a good source of vitamin C. When mixed with chamomile and mint and taken as a tea, it is an excellent way to help get a good night's sleep.

CHOCOLATE: Allow 1 small serving every other day. Keep them in your freezer so you know they are there to eat. Note the amount eaten. ___

CARBONATED BEVERAGES: Allow no more than 1 can. Enter amount consumed. ___

COFFEE: Allow no more than 3 cups today. Number of cups consumed today. ___

ALCOHOL: Allow no more than 3 drinks today. Write number consumed. ___

CIGARETTES: Try to smoke 5 or less cigarettes. Write number smoked today. ___

REFINED SUGARS: Limit sugars to 1 serving and white bread to 2 servings today. Enter number of servings consumed. ___

WATER: Drink 8 glasses of water. Note number of glasses. ___

Replace red meat with one of the following items. Check the item you picked.

beans ___	tofu ___	eggs ___	sprouts ___
almonds ___	TVP ___	cashews ___	chicken ___
turkey ___	lobster ___	salmon ___	tuna ___

EXERCISE: Walk briskly for 30 minutes without stopping. Check here when finished. ___

STRETCHING: Do exercise plan #2. Check here when finished. ___

SLEEP: Continue with ideas from back of workbook.

SUPPLEMENTS: Check here after taking your supplements. ___

ON A SCALE OF 1-10, with 1 indicating the least intensity, how you feel today? ___

JOURNAL OF HOW I FELT TODAY AND WHAT I ACCOMPLISHED

When going out to eat, it has been helpful for us to go to a buffet and eat a plate of fresh vegetables and fruit before going to the hot food bar. We also eat fewer foods that aren't so healthy since we are already partially full.

DAY 51

Catnip tea also helps relieve flatulence. (And that can be a relief to those around you!)

CHOCOLATE: Allow 1 small serving every other day. Keep them in your freezer so you know they are there to eat. Note the amount eaten. ___

CARBONATED BEVERAGES: Allow no more than 1 can. Enter amount consumed. ___

COFFEE: Allow no more than 3 cups today. Number of cups consumed today. ___

ALCOHOL: Allow no more than 3 drinks today. Write number consumed. ___

CIGARETTES: Try to smoke 5 or fewer cigarettes. Write number smoked today. ___

REFINED SUGARS: Limit sugars to 1 serving and white bread to 2 servings today. Enter number of servings consumed. ___

WATER: Drink 8 glasses of water. Note number of glasses. ___

Replace red meat with one of the following items. Check the item you picked.

beans	___	tofu	___	eggs	___	sprouts	___
almonds	___	TVP	___	cashews	___	chicken	___
turkey	___	lobster	___	salmon	___	tuna	___

EXERCISE: Walk briskly for 30 minutes without stopping. Check here when finished. ___

STRETCHING: Do exercise plan #3. Check here when finished. ___

SLEEP: Continue with ideas from back of workbook.

SUPPLEMENTS: Check here after taking your supplements. ___

ON A SCALE OF 1-10, with 1 indicating the least intensity, how you feel today? ___

JOURNAL OF HOW I FELT TODAY AND WHAT I ACCOMPLISHED

Supplements were an important part of getting better for us. We take a mineral supplement and a vitamin supplement daily.

DAY 52

Recently while talking to some women who had attended one of my programs the question was asked: "Do you really feel as good as you say you do?" My answer: "I feel better than I have in more than 20 years."

CHOCOLATE: Allow 1 small serving every other day. Keep them in your freezer so you know they are there to eat. Note the amount eaten. ____

CARBONATED BEVERAGES: Allow no more than 1 can. Enter amount consumed. ____

COFFEE: Allow no more than 3 cups today. Number of cups consumed today. ____

ALCOHOL: Allow no more than 3 drinks today. Write number consumed. ____

CIGARETTES: Try to smoke 5 or fewer cigarettes. Write number smoked today. ____

REFINED SUGARS: Limit sugars to 1 serving and white bread to 2 servings today. Enter number of servings consumed. ____

WATER: Drink 8 glasses of water. Note number of glasses. ____

Replace red meat with one of the following items. Check the item you picked.

beans	____	tofu	____	eggs	____	sprouts	____
almonds	____	TVP	____	cashews	____	chicken	____
turkey	____	lobster	____	salmon	____	tuna	____

EXERCISE: Walk briskly for 30 minutes without stopping. Check here when finished. ____

STRETCHING: Do exercise plan #1. Check here when finished. ____

SLEEP: Continue with ideas from back of workbook.

SUPPLEMENTS: Check here after taking your supplements. ____

ON A SCALE OF 1-10, with 1 indicating the least intensity, how you feel today? ____

JOURNAL OF HOW I FELT TODAY AND WHAT I ACCOMPLISHED

Kelly and I stay on a "maintenance program" to feel well most of the time. Once we started feeling well, and had felt well for more than a year, we found we could "cheat" once in a while. We don't cheat very often though, because after a couple of days we will start to notice pain making its way back into our bodies.

DAY 53

For years I thought everyone woke up every morning feeling like they had been beaten up during the night. I couldn't believe how wrong I was!

CHOCOLATE: Allow 1 small serving every other day. Keep them in your freezer so you know they are there to eat. Note the amount eaten.

CARBONATED BEVERAGES: Allow no more than 1 can. Enter amount consumed. ___

COFFEE: Allow no more than 3 cups today. Number of cups consumed today. ___

ALCOHOL: Allow no more than 3 drinks today. Write number consumed. ___

CIGARETTES: Try to smoke 5 or fewer cigarettes. Write number smoked today. ___

REFINED SUGARS: Limit sugars to 1 serving and white bread to 2 servings today. Enter number of servings consumed.

WATER: Drink 8 glasses of water. Note number of glasses. ___

Replace red meat with one of the following items. Check the item you picked.

beans	___	tofu	___	eggs	___	sprouts	___
almonds	___	TVP	___	cashews	___	chicken	___
turkey	___	lobster	___	salmon	___	tuna	___

EXERCISE: Walk briskly for 30 minutes without stopping. Check here when finished. ___

STRETCHING: Do exercise plan #1. Check here when finished. ___

SLEEP: Continue with ideas from back of workbook.

SUPPLEMENTS: Check here after taking your supplements. ___

ON A SCALE OF 1-10, with 1 indicating the least intensity, how you feel today? ___

JOURNAL OF HOW I FELT TODAY AND WHAT I ACCOMPLISHED

You too can feel better than you have in a long time. Keep working! By the way, one way to smooth the transition to eating healthier foods is to increase the amount of spices in your cooking.

DAY 54

With our bodies working less efficiently, toxins aren't released properly. It is believed this causes a toxic buildup in the tissues, which can also cause pain.

CHOCOLATE: Allow 1 small serving every other day. Keep them in your freezer so you know they are there to eat. Note the amount eaten. ——

CARBONATED BEVERAGES: Allow no more than 1 can. Enter amount consumed. ——

COFFEE: Allow no more than 3 cups today. Number of cups consumed today. ——

ALCOHOL: Allow no more than 3 drinks today. Write number consumed. ——

CIGARETTES: Try to smoke 5 or fewer cigarettes. Write number smoked today. ——

REFINED SUGARS: Limit sugars to 1 serving and white bread to 2 servings today. Enter number of servings consumed. ——

WATER: Drink 8 glasses of water. Note number of glasses. ——

Replace red meat with one of the following items. Check the item you picked.

beans	——	tofu	——	eggs	——	sprouts	——
almonds	——	TVP	——	cashews	——	chicken	——
turkey	——	lobster	——	salmon	——	tuna	——

EXERCISE: Walk briskly for 30 minutes without stopping. Check here when finished. ——

STRETCHING: Do exercise plan #2. Check here when finished. ——

SLEEP: Continue with ideas from back of workbook.

SUPPLEMENTS: Check here after taking your supplements. ——

ON A SCALE OF 1-10, with 1 indicating the least intensity, how you feel today? ——

JOURNAL OF HOW I FELT TODAY AND WHAT I ACCOMPLISHED

Any increase in physical exercise will help get muscles moving, which in turn helps the body to begin releasing toxins that are built up between tissues. This is one of the reasons exercise helps relieve pain.

DAY 55

Tight muscles can also create pain. If you notice tension or pain increasing in an area of your body, gently stretch that area.

CHOCOLATE: Allow 1 small serving every other day. Keep them in your freezer so you know they are there to eat. Note the amount eaten. ____

CARBONATED BEVERAGES: Allow no more than 1 can. Enter amount consumed. ____

COFFEE: Allow no more than 3 cups today. Number of cups consumed today. ____

ALCOHOL: Allow no more than 3 drinks today. Write number consumed. ____

CIGARETTES: Try to smoke 5 or fewer cigarettes. Write number smoked today. ____

REFINED SUGARS: Limit sugars to 1 serving and white bread to 2 servings today. Enter number of servings consumed. ____

WATER: Drink 8 glasses of water. Note number of glasses. ____

When omitting red meats from a meal, choose one of the following.

beans	____	tofu	____	eggs	____	sprouts	____
almonds	____	TVP	____	cashews	____	chicken	____
turkey	____	lobster	____	salmon	____	tuna	____

EXERCISE: Walk briskly for 30 minutes without stopping. Check here when finished. ____

STRETCHING: Do exercise plan #3. Check here when finished. ____

SLEEP: Continue with ideas from back of workbook.

SUPPLEMENTS: Check here after taking your supplements. ____

ON A SCALE OF 1-10, with 1 indicating the least intensity, how you feel today? ____

JOURNAL OF HOW I FELT TODAY AND WHAT I ACCOMPLISHED

Many of the exercises can be done at work, in a restroom or waiting room. Of course this doesn't include the exercises you have to get down on the floor to do!

DAY 56

Many times pain in the back of the head can be helped by massaging around the occipital bone at the lower base of the skull in the back of the head.

CHOCOLATE: Allow 1 small serving every other day. Keep them in your freezer so you know they are there to eat. Note the amount eaten. ___

CARBONATED BEVERAGES: Allow no more than 1 can. Enter amount consumed. ___

COFFEE: Allow no more than 3 cups today. Number of cups consumed today. ___

ALCOHOL: Allow no more than 3 drinks today. Write number consumed. ___

CIGARETTES: Try to smoke 5 or fewer cigarettes. Write number smoked today. ___

REFINED SUGARS: Limit sugars to 1 serving and white bread to 2 servings today. Enter number of servings consumed. ___

WATER: Drink 8 glasses of water. Note number of glasses. ___

When omitting red meats from a meal, choose one of the following.

beans ___	tofu ___	eggs ___	sprouts ___
almonds ___	TVP ___	cashews ___	chicken ___
turkey ___	lobster ___	salmon ___	tuna ___

EXERCISE: Walk briskly for 30 minutes without stopping. Check here when finished. ___

STRETCHING: Do exercise plan #1. Check here when finished. ___

SLEEP: Continue with ideas from back of workbook.

SUPPLEMENTS: Check here after taking your supplements. ___

ON A SCALE OF 1-10, with 1 indicating the least intensity, how you feel today? ___

JOURNAL OF HOW I FELT TODAY AND WHAT I ACCOMPLISHED

The area around the occipital bone may be very tender. Massaging will usually relieve the pressure, which may help relieve the headache pain.

DAY 57

It is believed by some that the areas of pain around the base of the occipital area in the head are related to organs within the body that are stressed.

CHOCOLATE: Allow 1 small serving every other day. Keep them in your freezer so you know they are there to eat. Note the amount eaten. ___

CARBONATED BEVERAGES: Allow no more than 1 can. Enter amount consumed. ___

COFFEE: Allow no more than 3 cups today. Number of cups consumed today. ___

ALCOHOL: Allow no more than 3 drinks today. Write number consumed. ___

CIGARETTES: Try to smoke 5 or fewer cigarettes. Write number smoked today. ___

REFINED SUGARS: Limit sugars to 1 serving and white bread to 2 servings today. Enter number of servings consumed. ___

WATER: Drink 8 glasses of water. Note number of glasses. ___

When omitting red meats from a meal, choose one of the following.

beans	___	tofu	___	eggs	___	sprouts	___
almonds	___	TVP	___	cashews	___	chicken	___
turkey	___	lobster	___	salmon	___	tuna	___

EXERCISE: Walk briskly for 30 minutes without stopping. Check here when finished. ___

STRETCHING: Do exercise plan #2. Check here when finished. ___

SLEEP: Continue with ideas from back of workbook.

SUPPLEMENTS: Check here after taking your supplements. ___

ON A SCALE OF 1-10, with 1 indicating the least intensity, how you feel today? ___

JOURNAL OF HOW I FELT TODAY AND WHAT I ACCOMPLISHED

Today in your journal list three areas of your life which are going poorly and three which are going well. Give yourself permission to worry about the three which are going poorly for about an hour. Once you've had a chance to worry about them, let them go and continue on with the day.

DAY 58

Our bodies need the proper food or "fuel" to run smoothly. If we put something other than gasoline into the gas tank of our car, we all know what would happen.

CHOCOLATE: Allow 1 small serving every other day. Keep them in your freezer so you know they are there to eat. Note the amount eaten. ____

CARBONATED BEVERAGES: Allow no more than 1 can. Enter amount consumed. ____

COFFEE: Allow no more than 3 cups today. Number of cups consumed today. ____

ALCOHOL: Allow no more than 3 drinks today. Write number consumed. ____

CIGARETTES: Try to smoke 5 or fewer cigarettes. Write number smoked today. ____

REFINED SUGARS: Limit sugars to 1 serving and white bread to 2 servings today. Enter number of servings consumed. ____

WATER: Drink 8 glasses of water. Note number of glasses. ____

When omitting red meats from a meal, choose one of the following.

beans	____	tofu	____	eggs	____	sprouts	____
almonds	____	TVP	____	cashews	____	chicken	____
turkey	____	lobster	____	salmon	____	tuna	____

EXERCISE: Walk briskly for 30 minutes without stopping. Check here when finished. ____

STRETCHING: Do exercise plan #3. Check here when finished. ____

SLEEP: Continue with ideas from back of workbook.

SUPPLEMENTS: Check here after taking your supplements. ____

ON A SCALE OF 1-10, with 1 indicating the least intensity, how you feel today? ____

JOURNAL OF HOW I FELT TODAY AND WHAT I ACCOMPLISHED

Help your body run better by making sure you put only the best sources of fuel in it!

DAY 59

Can you believe you have almost made it to the 2-month goal? By now you should be well into the program. Keep up the good work.

CHOCOLATE: Allow 1 small serving every other day. Keep them in your freezer so you know they are there to eat. Note the amount eaten.

CARBONATED BEVERAGES: Allow no more than 1 can. Enter amount consumed. ____

COFFEE: Allow no more than 3 cups today. Number of cups consumed today. ____

ALCOHOL: Allow no more than 3 drinks today. Write number consumed. ____

CIGARETTES: Try to smoke 5 or fewer cigarettes. Write number smoked today. ____

REFINED SUGARS: Limit sugars to 1 serving and white bread to 2 servings today. Enter number of servings consumed.

WATER: Drink 8 glasses of water. Note number of glasses. ____

When omitting red meats from a meal, choose one of the following.

beans	____	tofu	____	eggs	____	sprouts	____
almonds	____	TVP	____	cashews	____	chicken	____
turkey	____	lobster	____	salmon	____	tuna	____

EXERCISE: Walk briskly for 30 minutes without stopping. Check here when finished. ____

STRETCHING: Do exercise plan #1. Check here when finished. ____

SLEEP: Continue with ideas from back of workbook.

SUPPLEMENTS: Check here after taking your supplements. ____

ON A SCALE OF 1-10, with 1 indicating the least intensity, how you feel today? ____

JOURNAL OF HOW I FELT TODAY AND WHAT I ACCOMPLISHED

Remember, you didn't get this illness overnight. It will take a while to feel better. Keep working, if you slipped up on a few things or even a day, that's okay, just get back into the routine and you should start to feel better.

DAY 60!

Congratulations! You've made it through 2 months. From here on it should get easier. You have been making some drastic changes in your lifestyle. Keep working, because you'll be glad you did.

CHOCOLATE: Allow 1 serving 2 times a week. Note the amount eaten.   ——

CARBONATED BEVERAGES: Allow 1 can every other day. Enter amount consumed.   ——

COFFEE: Allow no more than 2 cups today. Number of cups consumed today.   ——

ALCOHOL: Allow no more than 2 drinks today. Write number consumed.   ——

CIGARETTES: Try to smoke 4 or fewer cigarettes. Write number smoked today.   ——

REFINED SUGARS: Limit sugars to 1 serving and white bread to 2 servings today. Enter number of servings consumed.   ——

WATER: Drink 8 glasses of water. Note number of glasses.   ——

When omitting red meats from a meal, choose one of the following.

beans	——	tofu	——	eggs	——	sprouts	——
almonds	——	TVP	——	cashews	——	chicken	——
turkey	——	lobster	——	salmon	——	tuna	——

EXERCISE: Walk briskly for 35 minutes without stopping. Check here when finished.   ——

STRETCHING: Do exercise plan #2. Check here when finished.   ——

SLEEP: Continue with ideas from back of workbook.

SUPPLEMENTS: Check here after taking your supplements.   ——

ON A SCALE OF 1-10, with 1 indicating the least intensity, how you feel today?   ——

JOURNAL OF HOW I FELT TODAY AND WHAT I ACCOMPLISHED

Remember that we are working only on lifestyle changes. Keep in mind that it takes 30 days to change a habit (and we are working on some very difficult habits to change). Be easy on yourself and follow the guide to help you with these changes. You're already half way through this book, so keep up the good work!

Congratulations!

You made it through 2 months. Go back to the beginning and read some of your entries to the journal. Compare those entries to the entries you are now making. Have there been any differences? If so, great! If not, the changes will come. Continue to thank your body for the healing process that is going on in it. You're doing positive things to improve the way you feel. It will pay off, so keep up the good work.

The Miracle

I saw a miracle today
as I was walking by.
It wasn't on the ground or in the water
but rather in the sky.
And as I watched this miracle
my heart would leap in joy;
That such a wonder could come my way,
In the middle of the day.
This miracle high up in the sky
was playing like a child.
Actually not one or two or three or four
But many birds from the wild.
As they flew up in the distance
And turned and whirled and traveled
Their wings would glisten then disappear
then turn black as the picture unraveled.
This wonderful miracle I watched in awe
For maybe five or ten minutes.
Enjoying nature's gift to me that day
As in my world they played.
Then as quickly as they came they also disappeared.
On their way to who knows where
As the sky I watched was cleared.
I thank the earth for her gifts of beauty
And am thankful that on this day,
She brought the flock into my view
To play for me their wondrous show.
Then just as quickly disappeared as on our paths we go.

Mary Moeller

Health Evaluation Form

Refer back to this page only one time per month; after you have filled out the HEF for the next month.

Indicate in the column next to the symptoms which of the following conditions apply to you in terms of frequency and/or intensity of symptoms using the numbers 1-10: 1 being the least amount of intensity and 10 being the greatest. After filling it out, refer to the HEF form filled out in the front section of the workbook to compare the differences.

Low energy/Often feel tired		Light sleep/aware of surroundings	
Skin problems–dry, itchy, acne		Cold hands and feet	
Headaches/migraines		Shortness of breath	
Aching joints		Often feel bloated	
Muscle cramps		Bowel gas	
Menstrual cramps/moody/PMS			
Cuts and bruises heal slowly		Heartburn/indigestion	
Poor concentration		Constipation/diarrhea	
Difficulty handling stress		Weak fingernails/Unhealthy hair	
Strong desire for sweets/salts		Poor muscle tone	
High/low blood pressure		Water retention	
Frequently take pain killers		Cellulite	
Moods of depression		Allergies/Hayfever	
Difficulty getting up in morning		Poor night vision	
Difficulty falling asleep		Varicose veins	
		Hemorrhoids	

How many glasses of water do you drink each day? ____
How many cups of coffee do you drink each day? ____
How many times do you drink alcohol each day? ____
How many cans of pop do you drink each day? ____
How many times do you eat chocolate each day? ____
How many times do you eat red meat each day? ____
How much weight have you gained in the past year? ____

DAY 61

We will make a few more changes this month, so be sure to read through each area carefully.

CHOCOLATE: Allow 1 serving 2 times a week. Note the amount eaten. ___

CARBONATED BEVERAGES: Allow 1 can every other day. Enter amount consumed. ___

COFFEE: Allow no more than 2 cups today. Number of cups consumed today. ___

ALCOHOL: Allow no more than 1 drink every other day. Write number consumed. ___

CIGARETTES: Try to smoke 4 or fewer cigarettes. Write number smoked today. ___

REFINED SUGARS: Limit sugars to every other day and white bread to 2 servings a day. Enter number of servings consumed. ___

WATER: Drink 8 glasses of water. Note number of glasses. ___

When omitting red meats from a meal, choose one of the following.

beans	___	tofu	___	eggs	___	sprouts	___
almonds	___	TVP	___	cashews	___	chicken	___
turkey	___	lobster	___	salmon	___	tuna	___

EXERCISE: Walk briskly for 35 minutes without stopping. Check here when finished. ___

STRETCHING: Do exercise plan #1. Check here when finished. ___

SLEEP: Continue with ideas from back of workbook.

SUPPLEMENTS: Check here after taking your supplements. ___

ON A SCALE OF 1-10, with 1 indicating the least intensity, how you feel today? ___

JOURNAL OF HOW I FELT TODAY AND WHAT I ACCOMPLISHED

As the program continues, we will try to eliminate from your diet these foods: chocolate, coffee, carbonated beverages and alcohol. We will also try to decrease the amount of sugars consumed.

DAY 62

Okay, so you're getting a little tired of this old drag of watching everything that goes into your mouth. I know the feeling, but don't forget that most of us who feel good have been through it.

CHOCOLATE: Allow 1 serving 2 times a week. Note the amount eaten.   ——

CARBONATED BEVERAGES: Allow 1 can every other day. Enter amount consumed.   ——

COFFEE: Allow no more than 2 cups today. Number of cups consumed today.   ——

ALCOHOL: Allow no more than 1 drink every other day. Write number consumed.   ——

CIGARETTES: Try to smoke 4 or fewer cigarettes. Write number smoked today.   ——

REFINED SUGARS: Limit sugars to every other day and white bread to 2 servings a day. Enter number of servings consumed.   ——

WATER: Drink 8 glasses of water. Note number of glasses.   ——

When omitting red meats from a meal, choose one of the following.

beans	——	tofu	——	eggs	——	sprouts	——
almonds	——	TVP	——	cashews	——	chicken	——
turkey	——	lobster	——	salmon	——	tuna	——

EXERCISE: Walk briskly for 35 minutes without stopping. Check here when finished.   ——

STRETCHING: Do exercise plan #2. Check here when finished.   ——

SLEEP: Continue with ideas from back of workbook.

SUPPLEMENTS: Check here after taking your supplements.   ——

ON A SCALE OF 1-10, with 1 indicating the least intensity, how you feel today?   ——

JOURNAL OF HOW I FELT TODAY AND WHAT I ACCOMPLISHED

Remember to drink a small glass of juice or have a small piece of fruit every 2 hours to avoid the sugar cravings. It has worked great for me.

DAY 63

Remember that you didn't get this sickness overnight. You've probably had some of many of the symptoms for a long time. It will take a while for your body to heal itself.

CHOCOLATE: Allow 1 serving 2 times a week. Note the amount eaten. _____
CARBONATED BEVERAGES: Allow 1 can every other day. Enter amount consumed. _____
COFFEE: Allow no more than 2 cups today. Number of cups consumed today. _____
ALCOHOL: Allow no more than 1 drink every other day. Write number consumed. _____
CIGARETTES: Try to smoke 4 or fewer cigarettes. Write number smoked today. _____
REFINED SUGARS: Limit sugars to every other day and white bread to 2 servings a day.
   Enter number of servings consumed. _____
WATER: Drink 8 glasses of water. Note number of glasses. _____

When omitting red meats from a meal, choose one of the following.

beans	_____	tofu	_____	eggs	_____	sprouts	_____
almonds	_____	TVP	_____	cashews	_____	chicken	_____
turkey	_____	lobster	_____	salmon	_____	tuna	_____

EXERCISE: Walk briskly for 35 minutes without stopping. Check here when finished. _____
STRETCHING: Do exercise plan #3. Check here when finished. _____
SLEEP: Continue with ideas from back of workbook.
SUPPLEMENTS: Check here after taking your supplements. _____
ON A SCALE OF 1-10, with 1 indicating the least intensity, how you feel today? _____

JOURNAL OF HOW I FELT TODAY AND WHAT I ACCOMPLISHED

As you may have already found out, medications may help one or two symptoms, but it is difficult to find a medications that will take care of all your symptoms. The changes we make to feel better take time, persistence and a lot of work, but it's worth every bit of the work to feel well again.

DAY 64

Supplements were very important for Kelly and my recovery. Be sure to use quality supplements. I have very poor results when using the generic brands.

CHOCOLATE: Allow 1 serving 2 times a week. Note the amount eaten. ___
CARBONATED BEVERAGES: Allow 1 can every other day. Enter amount consumed. ___
COFFEE: Allow no more than 2 cups today. Number of cups consumed today. ___
ALCOHOL: Allow no more than 1 drink every other day. Write number consumed. ___
CIGARETTES: Try to smoke 4 or fewer cigarettes. Write number smoked today. ___
REFINED SUGARS: Limit sugars to every other day and white bread to 2 servings a day.
 Enter number of servings consumed. ___
WATER: Drink 8 glasses of water. Note number of glasses. ___

When omitting red meats from a meal, choose one of the following.

beans	___	tofu	___	eggs	___	sprouts	___
almonds	___	TVP	___	cashews	___	chicken	___
turkey	___	lobster	___	salmon	___	tuna	___

EXERCISE: Walk briskly for 35 minutes without stopping. Check here when finished. ___
STRETCHING: Do exercise plan #1. Check here when finished. ___
SLEEP: Continue with ideas from back of workbook.
SUPPLEMENTS: Check here after taking your supplements. ___
ON A SCALE OF 1-10, with 1 indicating the least intensity, how you feel today? ___

JOURNAL OF HOW I FELT TODAY AND WHAT I ACCOMPLISHED

You may need to try a number of different brands of supplements before you find one that helps. You should be able to detect some difference in energy level within 4-6 weeks if the supplement is good for you.

DAY 65

Mineral supplements have been an important addition to my diet.

CHOCOLATE: Allow 1 serving 2 times a week. Note the amount eaten. ___
CARBONATED BEVERAGES: Allow 1 can every other day. Enter amount consumed. ___
COFFEE: Allow no more than 2 cups today. Number of cups consumed today. ___
ALCOHOL: Allow no more than 1 drink every other day. Write number consumed. ___
CIGARETTES: Try to smoke 4 or fewer cigarettes. Write number smoked today. ___
REFINED SUGARS: Limit sugars to every other day and white bread to 2 servings a day. Enter number of servings consumed.
WATER: Drink 8 glasses of water. Note number of glasses. ___

When omitting red meats from a meal, choose one of the following.

beans ___	tofu ___	eggs ___	sprouts ___
almonds ___	TVP ___	cashews ___	chicken ___
turkey ___	lobster ___	salmon ___	tuna ___

EXERCISE: Walk briskly for 35 minutes without stopping. Check here when finished. ___
STRETCHING: Do exercise plan #2. Check here when finished. ___
SLEEP: Continue with ideas from back of workbook.
SUPPLEMENTS: Check here after taking your supplements. ___
ON A SCALE OF 1-10, with 1 indicating the least intensity, how you feel today? ___

JOURNAL OF HOW I FELT TODAY AND WHAT I ACCOMPLISHED

I always take my mineral supplements with food to avoid an upset stomach.

DAY 66

Parsley is very nutritious and makes a pretty plant for flower beds. One to two handfuls of fresh parsley eaten daily can provide a hearty dose of many vitamins and minerals, including calcium.

CHOCOLATE: Allow 1 serving 2 times a week. Note the amount eaten. ____

CARBONATED BEVERAGES: Allow 1 can every other day. Enter amount consumed. ____

COFFEE: Allow no more than 2 cups today. Number of cups consumed today. ____

ALCOHOL: Allow no more than 1 drink every other day. Write number consumed. ____

CIGARETTES: Try to smoke 4 or fewer cigarettes. Write number smoked today. ____

REFINED SUGARS: Limit sugars to every other day and white bread to 2 servings a day. Enter number of servings consumed. ____

WATER: Drink 8 glasses of water. Note number of glasses. ____

When omitting red meats from a meal, choose one of the following.

beans	____	tofu	____	eggs	____	sprouts	____
almonds	____	TVP	____	cashews	____	chicken	____
turkey	____	lobster	____	salmon	____	tuna	____

EXERCISE: Walk briskly for 35 minutes without stopping. Check here when finished. ____

STRETCHING: Do exercise plan #2. Check here when finished. ____

SLEEP: Continue with ideas from back of workbook.

SUPPLEMENTS: Check here after taking your supplements. ____

ON A SCALE OF 1-10, with 1 indicating the least intensity, how you feel today? ____

JOURNAL OF HOW I FELT TODAY AND WHAT I ACCOMPLISHED

If left to flower, parsley will reseed itself and will come up the following year. I need to replant parsley in my garden about once every four years.

DAY 67

Parsley has been used as a diuretic and liver tonic to break up kidney stones and to soothe coughs.

CHOCOLATE: Allow 1 serving 2 times a week. Note the amount eaten. ___
CARBONATED BEVERAGES: Allow 1 can every other day. Enter amount consumed. ___
COFFEE: Allow no more than 2 cups today. Number of cups consumed today. ___
ALCOHOL: Allow no more than 1 drink every other day. Write number consumed. ___
CIGARETTES: Try to smoke 4 or fewer cigarettes. Write number smoked today. ___
REFINED SUGARS: Limit sugars to every other day and white bread to 2 servings a day. Enter number of servings consumed. ___
WATER: Drink 8 glasses of water. Note number of glasses. ___

When omitting red meats from a meal, choose one of the following.

beans ___	tofu ___	eggs ___	sprouts ___
almonds ___	TVP ___	cashews ___	chicken ___
turkey ___	lobster ___	salmon ___	tuna ___

EXERCISE: Walk briskly for 35 minutes without stopping. Check here when finished. ___
STRETCHING: Do exercise plan #3. Check here when finished. ___
SLEEP: Continue with ideas from back of workbook.
SUPPLEMENTS: Check here after taking your supplements. ___
ON A SCALE OF 1-10, with 1 indicating the least intensity, how you feel today? ___

JOURNAL OF HOW I FELT TODAY AND WHAT I ACCOMPLISHED

Parsley is a good addition to diets for people who have problems with anemia.

DAY 68

Keep in mind that too much fresh parsley can irritate the kidneys.

CHOCOLATE: Allow 1 serving 2 times a week. Note the amount eaten. ___

CARBONATED BEVERAGES: Allow 1 can every other day. Enter amount consumed. ___

COFFEE: Allow no more than 2 cups today. Number of cups consumed today. ___

ALCOHOL: Allow no more than 1 drink every other day. Write number consumed. ___

CIGARETTES: Try to smoke 4 or fewer cigarettes. Write number smoked today. ___

REFINED SUGARS: Limit sugars to every other day and white bread to 2 servings a day.
Enter number of servings consumed. ___

WATER: Drink 8 glasses of water. Note number of glasses. ___

When omitting red meats from a meal, choose one of the following.

beans	___	tofu	___	eggs	___	sprouts	___
almonds	___	TVP	___	cashews	___	chicken	___
turkey	___	lobster	___	salmon	___	tuna	___

EXERCISE: Walk briskly for 35 minutes without stopping. Check here when finished. ___

STRETCHING: Do exercise plan #1. Check here when finished. ___

SLEEP: Continue with ideas from back of workbook.

SUPPLEMENTS: Check here after taking your supplements. ___

ON A SCALE OF 1-10, with 1 indicating the least intensity, how you feel today? ___

JOURNAL OF HOW I FELT TODAY AND WHAT I ACCOMPLISHED

Eat no more than 2 handfuls of parsley a day.

DAY 69

It is important to eat as many fresh fruits and vegetables as possible.

CHOCOLATE: Allow 1 serving 2 times a week. Note the amount eaten. ___
CARBONATED BEVERAGES: Allow 1 can every other day. Enter amount consumed. ___
COFFEE: Allow no more than 2 cups today. Number of cups consumed today. ___
ALCOHOL: Allow no more than 1 drink every other day. Write number consumed. ___
CIGARETTES: Try to smoke 4 or fewer cigarettes. Write number smoked today. ___
REFINED SUGARS: Limit sugars to every other day and white bread to 2 servings a day.
Enter number of servings consumed. ___
WATER: Drink 8 glasses of water. Note number of glasses. ___

When omitting red meats from a meal, choose one of the following.

beans	___	tofu	___	eggs	___	sprouts	___
almonds	___	TVP	___	cashews	___	chicken	___
turkey	___	lobster	___	salmon	___	tuna	___

EXERCISE: Walk briskly for 35 minutes without stopping. Check here when finished. ___
STRETCHING: Do exercise plan #2. Check here when finished. ___
SLEEP: Continue with ideas from back of workbook.
SUPPLEMENTS: Check here after taking your supplements. ___
ON A SCALE OF 1-10, with 1 indicating the least intensity, how you feel today? ___

JOURNAL OF HOW I FELT TODAY AND WHAT I ACCOMPLISHED

Start eating more fresh fruits and vegetables, increasing consumption to 40 percent of all food you eat.

DAY 70

Since our bodies many times don't metabolize foods as efficiently as they should or could, the amount of nutrients we receive from the food we eat could be much less than a person without FMS.

CHOCOLATE: Allow 1 serving 2 times a week. Note the amount eaten. ____

CARBONATED BEVERAGES: Allow 1 can every other day. Enter amount consumed. ____

COFFEE: Allow no more than 2 cups today. Number of cups consumed today. ____

ALCOHOL: Allow no more than 1 drink every other day. Write number consumed. ____

CIGARETTES: Try to smoke 4 or fewer cigarettes. Write number smoked today. ____

REFINED SUGARS: Limit sugars to every other day and white bread to 2 servings a day. Enter number of servings consumed. ____

WATER: Drink 8 glasses of water. Note number of glasses. ____

Replace red meat with one of the following.

beans	____	tofu	____	eggs	____	sprouts	____
almonds	____	TVP	____	cashews	____	chicken	____
turkey	____	lobster	____	salmon	____	tuna	____

EXERCISE: Walk briskly for 35 minutes without stopping. Check here when finished. ____

STRETCHING: Do exercise plan #3. Check here when finished. ____

SLEEP: Continue with ideas from back of workbook.

SUPPLEMENTS: Check here after taking your supplements. ____

ON A SCALE OF 1-10, with 1 indicating the least intensity, how you feel today? ____

JOURNAL OF HOW I FELT TODAY AND WHAT I ACCOMPLISHED

When we eat foods that have been cooked, many of the nutrients are lost due to the cooking process. Since our bodies may not utilize the nutrients in our foods as well as healthy bodies, we are probably getting even fewer nutrients from cooked foods than a healthy person would get.

DAY 71

Once I started eating more fresh fruits and vegetables, I noticed an increase in energy levels.

CHOCOLATE: Allow 1 serving 2 times a week. Note the amount eaten. ___
CARBONATED BEVERAGES: Allow 1 can every other day. Enter amount consumed. ___
COFFEE: Allow no more than 2 cups today. Number of cups consumed today. ___
ALCOHOL: Allow no more than 1 drink every other day. Write number consumed. ___
CIGARETTES: Try to smoke 4 or fewer cigarettes. Write number smoked today. ___
REFINED SUGARS: Limit sugars to every other day and white bread to 2 servings a day.
Enter number of servings consumed. ___
WATER: Drink 8 glasses of water. Note number of glasses. ___

Replace red meat with one of the following.

beans	___	tofu	___	eggs	___	sprouts	___
almonds	___	TVP	___	cashews	___	chicken	___
turkey	___	lobster	___	salmon	___	tuna	___

EXERCISE: Walk briskly for 35 minutes without stopping. Check here when finished. ___
STRETCHING: Do exercise plan #1. Check here when finished. ___
SLEEP: Continue with ideas from back of workbook.
SUPPLEMENTS: Check here after taking your supplements. ___
ON A SCALE OF 1-10, with 1 indicating the least intensity, how you feel today? ___

JOURNAL OF HOW I FELT TODAY AND WHAT I ACCOMPLISHED

Regardless of the time of year, start trying new "summer" recipes, which usually include more fresh ingredients.

DAY 72

To make a fast, easy, accessible meal, try mixing broccoli, cauliflower, carrots, peppers and celery in a food processor. Keep the salad in the freezer or refrigerator until you want to use it. Put you favorite dressing on it for a flavorful, healthy diet.

CHOCOLATE: Allow 1 serving 2 times a week. Note the amount eaten. ___
CARBONATED BEVERAGES: Allow 1 can every other day. Enter amount consumed. ___
COFFEE: Allow no more than 2 cups today. Number of cups consumed today. ___
ALCOHOL: Allow no more than 1 drink every other day. Write number consumed. ___
CIGARETTES: Try to smoke 4 or fewer cigarettes. Write number smoked today. ___
REFINED SUGARS: Limit sugars to every other day and white bread to 2 servings a day. Enter number of servings consumed. ___
WATER: Drink 8 glasses of water. Note number of glasses. ___

Replace red meat with one of the following.

beans ___	tofu ___	eggs ___	sprouts ___
almonds ___	TVP ___	cashews ___	chicken ___
turkey ___	lobster ___	salmon ___	tuna ___

EXERCISE: Walk briskly for 35 minutes without stopping. Check here when finished. ___
STRETCHING: Do exercise plan #1. Check here when finished. ___
SLEEP: Continue with ideas from back of workbook.
SUPPLEMENTS: Check here after taking your supplements. ___
ON A SCALE OF 1-10, with 1 indicating the least intensity, how you feel today? ___

JOURNAL OF HOW I FELT TODAY AND WHAT I ACCOMPLISHED

These vegetables are also good on top of lettuce or in soup.

DAY 73

Garlic is a wonderful herb to add to your diet and garden.

CHOCOLATE: Allow 1 serving 2 times a week. Note the amount eaten. ___
CARBONATED BEVERAGES: Allow 1 can every other day. Enter amount consumed. ___
COFFEE: Allow no more than 2 cups today. Number of cups consumed today. ___
ALCOHOL: Allow no more than 1 drink every other day. Write number consumed. ___
CIGARETTES: Try to smoke 4 or fewer cigarettes. Write number smoked today. ___
REFINED SUGARS: Limit sugars to every other day and white bread to 2 servings a day.
Enter number of servings consumed. ___
WATER: Drink 8 glasses of water. Note number of glasses. ___

Replace red meat with one of the following.

beans ___	tofu ___	eggs ___	sprouts ___
almonds ___	TVP ___	cashews ___	chicken ___
turkey ___	lobster ___	salmon ___	tuna ___

EXERCISE: Walk briskly for 35 minutes without stopping. Check here when finished. ___
STRETCHING: Do exercise plan #2. Check here when finished. ___
SLEEP: Continue with ideas from back of workbook.
SUPPLEMENTS: Check here after taking your supplements. ___
ON A SCALE OF 1-10, with 1 indicating the least intensity, how you feel today? ___

JOURNAL OF HOW I FELT TODAY AND WHAT I ACCOMPLISHED

Garlic has an old reputation of helping to lower blood pressure.

DAY 74

If your symptoms of pain are caused from Candida (yeast) overgrowth, there are a number of natural remedies that may be of help. Garlic is one of the herbs that help get rid of Candida.

CHOCOLATE: Allow 1 serving 2 times a week. Note the amount eaten.   ___

CARBONATED BEVERAGES: Allow 1 can every other day. Enter amount consumed.   ___

COFFEE: Allow no more than 2 cups today. Number of cups consumed today.   ___

ALCOHOL: Allow no more than 1 drink every other day. Write number consumed.   ___

CIGARETTES: Try to smoke 4 or fewer cigarettes. Write number smoked today.   ___

REFINED SUGARS: Limit sugars to every other day and white bread to 2 servings a day. Enter number of servings consumed.   ___

WATER: Drink 8 glasses of water. Note number of glasses.   ___

Replace red meat with one of the following.

beans	___	tofu	___	eggs	___	sprouts	___
almonds	___	TVP	___	cashews	___	chicken	___
turkey	___	lobster	___	salmon	___	tuna	___

EXERCISE: Walk briskly for 35 minutes without stopping. Check here when finished.   ___

STRETCHING: Do exercise plan #3. Check here when finished.   ___

SLEEP: Continue with ideas from back of workbook.

SUPPLEMENTS: Check here after taking your supplements.   ___

ON A SCALE OF 1-10, with 1 indicating the least intensity, how you feel today?   ___

JOURNAL OF HOW I FELT TODAY AND WHAT I ACCOMPLISHED

I have added garlic to much of my cooking, and have found it to be a wonderful addition to my recipes.

DAY 75

Garlic planted around fruit and nut trees will help keep moles away.

CHOCOLATE: Allow 1 serving 2 times a week. Note the amount eaten.
CARBONATED BEVERAGES: Allow 1 can every other day. Enter amount consumed. ___
COFFEE: Allow no more than 2 cups today. Number of cups consumed today. ___
ALCOHOL: Allow no more than 1 drink every other day. Write number consumed. ___
CIGARETTES: Try to smoke 4 or fewer cigarettes. Write number smoked today. ___
REFINED SUGARS: Limit sugars to every other day and white bread to 2 servings a day.
Enter number of servings consumed. ___
WATER: Drink 8 glasses of water. Note number of glasses. ___

Replace red meat with one of the following.

beans	___	tofu	___	eggs	___	sprouts	___
almonds	___	TVP	___	cashews	___	chicken	___
turkey	___	lobster	___	salmon	___	tuna	___

EXERCISE: Walk briskly for 35 minutes without stopping. Check here when finished. ___
STRETCHING: Do exercise plan #1. Check here when finished. ___
SLEEP: Continue with ideas from back of workbook.
SUPPLEMENTS: Check here after taking your supplements. ___
ON A SCALE OF 1-10, with 1 indicating the least intensity, how you feel today? ___

JOURNAL OF HOW I FELT TODAY AND WHAT I ACCOMPLISHED

Planted around rose bushes, garlic will help repel aphids.

DAY 76

A couple of years ago, I noticed some ants that had made their way into our home via a small crack in the window sill. Garlic worked wonders in keeping them at bay.

CHOCOLATE: Allow 1 serving 2 times a week. Note the amount eaten. ___

CARBONATED BEVERAGES: Allow 1 can every other day. Enter amount consumed. ___

COFFEE: Allow no more than 2 cups today. Number of cups consumed today. ___

ALCOHOL: Allow no more than 1 drink every other day. Write number consumed. ___

CIGARETTES: Try to smoke 4 or fewer cigarettes. Write number smoked today. ___

REFINED SUGARS: Limit sugars to every other day and white bread to 2 servings a day. Enter number of servings consumed. ___

WATER: Drink 8 glasses of water. Note number of glasses. ___

Replace red meat with one of the following.

beans	___	tofu	___	eggs	___	sprouts	___
almonds	___	TVP	___	cashews	___	chicken	___
turkey	___	lobster	___	salmon	___	tuna	___

EXERCISE: Walk briskly for 35 minutes without stopping. Check here when finished. ___

STRETCHING: Do exercise plan #2. Check here when finished. ___

SLEEP: Continue with ideas from back of workbook.

SUPPLEMENTS: Check here after taking your supplements. ___

ON A SCALE OF 1-10, with 1 indicating the least intensity, how you feel today? ___

JOURNAL OF HOW I FELT TODAY AND WHAT I ACCOMPLISHED

I pour some garlic tea in my window sills to keep black ants away. You may not want to pour the tea in your window sills if you don't have an area for the tea to drain out of the sills.

DAY 77

A wonderful way to use garlic to enhance spaghetti, noodles, etc., is to saute fresh garlic and parsley in two tablespoons of olive oil. Toss the spaghetti in the oil mixture.

CHOCOLATE: Allow 1 serving 2 times a week. Note the amount eaten. ___

CARBONATED BEVERAGES: Allow 1 can every other day. Enter amount consumed. ___

COFFEE: Allow no more than 2 cups today. Number of cups consumed today. ___

ALCOHOL: Allow no more than 1 drink every other day. Write number consumed. ___

CIGARETTES: Try to smoke 4 or fewer cigarettes. Write number smoked today. ___

REFINED SUGARS: Limit sugars to every other day and white bread to 2 servings a day. Enter number of servings consumed. ___

WATER: Drink 8 glasses of water. Note number of glasses. ___

Replace red meat with one of the following.

beans	___	tofu	___	eggs	___	sprouts	___
almonds	___	TVP	___	cashews	___	chicken	___
turkey	___	lobster	___	salmon	___	tuna	___

EXERCISE: Walk briskly for 35 minutes without stopping. Check here when finished. ___

STRETCHING: Do exercise plan #3. Check here when finished. ___

SLEEP: Continue with ideas from back of workbook.

SUPPLEMENTS: Check here after taking your supplements. ___

ON A SCALE OF 1-10, with 1 indicating the least intensity, how you feel today? ___

JOURNAL OF HOW I FELT TODAY AND WHAT I ACCOMPLISHED

The spaghetti can be eaten that way or doused in spaghetti sauce.

DAY 78

You're doing well. If you've slipped a little, give yourself a break. You can always start fresh again tomorrow.

CHOCOLATE: Allow 1 serving 2 times a week. Note the amount eaten.   ____

CARBONATED BEVERAGES: Allow 1 can every other day. Enter amount consumed.   ____

COFFEE: Allow no more than 2 cups today. Number of cups consumed today.   ____

ALCOHOL: Allow no more than 1 drink every other day. Write number consumed.   ____

CIGARETTES: Try to smoke 4 or fewer cigarettes. Write number smoked today.   ____

REFINED SUGARS: Limit sugars to every other day and white bread to 2 servings a day. Enter number of servings consumed.   ____

WATER: Drink 8 glasses of water. Note number of glasses.   ____

Replace red meat with one of the following.

beans	___	tofu	___	eggs	___	sprouts	___
almonds	___	TVP	___	cashews	___	chicken	___
turkey	___	lobster	___	salmon	___	tuna	___

EXERCISE: Walk briskly for 35 minutes without stopping. Check here when finished.   ____

STRETCHING: Do exercise plan #1. Check here when finished.   ____

SLEEP: Continue with ideas from back of workbook.

SUPPLEMENTS: Check here after taking your supplements.   ____

ON A SCALE OF 1-10, with 1 indicating the least intensity, how you feel today?   ____

JOURNAL OF HOW I FELT TODAY AND WHAT I ACCOMPLISHED

You are almost 3 months into the program. If you aren't already noticing improvements, you soon should!

DAY 79

Remember that the goal is to eliminate completely from our diets the following: chocolate, carbonated beverages, coffee, alcohol and cigarettes.

CHOCOLATE: Allow 1 serving 2 times a week. Note the amount eaten. ___

CARBONATED BEVERAGES: Allow 1 can every other day. Enter amount consumed. ___

COFFEE: Allow no more than 2 cups today. Number of cups consumed today. ___

ALCOHOL: Allow no more than 1 drink every other day. Write number consumed. ___

CIGARETTES: Try to smoke 4 or fewer cigarettes. Write number smoked today. ___

REFINED SUGARS: Limit sugars to every other day and white bread to 2 servings a day. Enter number of servings consumed. ___

WATER: Drink 8 glasses of water. Note number of glasses. ___

Replace red meat with one of the following.

beans	___	tofu	___	eggs	___	sprouts	___
almonds	___	TVP	___	cashews	___	chicken	___
turkey	___	lobster	___	salmon	___	tuna	___

EXERCISE: Walk briskly for 35 minutes without stopping. Check here when finished. ___

STRETCHING: Do exercise plan #2. Check here when finished. ___

SLEEP: Continue with ideas from back of workbook.

SUPPLEMENTS: Check here after taking your supplements. ___

ON A SCALE OF 1-10, with 1 indicating the least intensity, how you feel today? ___

JOURNAL OF HOW I FELT TODAY AND WHAT I ACCOMPLISHED

Many times people tell me that if they must eat so healthy, they just as well not be alive because life isn't worth living if a person has to give up all the "good" things in life to feel well. Once I changed my attitude and focus, a noticeable physical healing began to take place. I would rather enjoy the hours of fun and be able to do everything else I had wanted to do for so long, but didn't fell well enough to do, than worry about 20 minutes of food three times a day. What do you think?

DAY 80

I am very careful to watch the MSG preservative in foods. Many of your canned soups contain MSG.

CHOCOLATE: Allow 1 serving 2 times a week. Note the amount eaten. ___

CARBONATED BEVERAGES: Allow 1 can every other day. Enter amount consumed. ___

COFFEE: Allow no more than 2 cups today. Number of cups consumed today. ___

ALCOHOL: Allow no more than 1 drink every other day. Write number consumed. ___

CIGARETTES: Try to smoke 4 or fewer cigarettes. Write number smoked today. ___

REFINED SUGARS: Limit sugars to every other day and white bread to 2 servings a day. Enter number of servings consumed. ___

WATER: Drink 8 glasses of water. Note number of glasses. ___

Replace red meat with one of the following.

beans	___	tofu	___	eggs	___	sprouts	___
almonds	___	TVP	___	cashews	___	chicken	___
turkey	___	lobster	___	salmon	___	tuna	___

EXERCISE: Walk briskly for 35 minutes without stopping. Check here when finished. ___

STRETCHING: Do exercise plan #3. Check here when finished. ___

SLEEP: Continue with ideas from back of workbook.

SUPPLEMENTS: Check here after taking your supplements. ___

ON A SCALE OF 1-10, with 1 indicating the least intensity, how you feel today? ___

JOURNAL OF HOW I FELT TODAY AND WHAT I ACCOMPLISHED

Be sure to check labels of soup products to be sure there is no MSG present.

DAY 81

Recently we took a trip to Branson, Missouri, and while there we went into a store in a mall. In this store were about 10 people handing out samples of snack foods to customers as they walked in the door. Within 25 minutes after walking into the door of that store I had a horrible headache.

CHOCOLATE: Allow 1 serving 2 times a week. Note the amount eaten. ___
CARBONATED BEVERAGES: Allow 1 can every 3 days. Drink less if possible.
Enter amount consumed. ___
COFFEE: Allow no more than 1 cup today. Number of cups consumed today. ___
ALCOHOL: Allow no more than 1 drink every 3 days. Write number consumed. ___
CIGARETTES: Try to smoke 4 or fewer cigarettes. Write number smoked today. ___
REFINED SUGARS: Limit sugars to twice a week and breads and pastas to 3 servings.
Enter number of servings consumed. ___
WATER: Drink 8 glasses of water. Note number of glasses. ___

Replace red meat with one of the following.

beans	___	tofu	___	eggs	___	sprouts	___
almonds	___	TVP	___	cashews	___	chicken	___
turkey	___	lobster	___	salmon	___	tuna	___

EXERCISE: Walk briskly for 35 minutes without stopping. Check here when finished. ___
STRETCHING: Do exercise plan #2. Check here when finished. ___
SLEEP: Continue with ideas from back of workbook.
SUPPLEMENTS: Check here after taking your supplements. ___
ON A SCALE OF 1-10, with 1 indicating the least intensity, how you feel today? ___

JOURNAL OF HOW I FELT TODAY AND WHAT I ACCOMPLISHED

Aspirin didn't faze this headache, so I had to go back to the motel and do a massage treatment on my legs to get rid of the headache. The massage treatment can be found in the back of the book in the reference section.

DAY 82

Once again I would like to accentuate the necessity of minerals in my diet. As I said earlier, there are some minerals that people with FMS seem to be deficient in. Those are magnesium, manganese, folic acid, B vitamins, zinc calcium and vitamin C.

CHOCOLATE: Allow 1 serving 2 times a week. Note the amount eaten. ___

CARBONATED BEVERAGES: Allow 1 can every 3 days. Drink less if possible.
Enter amount consumed. ___

COFFEE: Allow no more than 1 cup today. Number of cups consumed today. ___

ALCOHOL: Allow no more than 1 drink every 3 days. Write number consumed. ___

CIGARETTES: Try to smoke 3 or fewer cigarettes. Write number smoked today. ___

REFINED SUGARS: Limit sugars to twice a week and breads and pastas to 3 servings.
Enter number of servings consumed. ___

WATER: Drink 8 glasses of water. Note number of glasses. ___

Replace red meat with one of the following.

beans	___	tofu	___	eggs	___	sprouts	___
almonds	___	TVP	___	cashews	___	chicken	___
turkey	___	lobster	___	salmon	___	tuna	___

EXERCISE: Walk briskly for 35 minutes without stopping. Check here when finished. ___

STRETCHING: Do exercise plan #3. Check here when finished. ___

SLEEP: Continue with ideas from back of workbook.

SUPPLEMENTS: Check here after taking your supplements. ___

ON A SCALE OF 1-10, with 1 indicating the least intensity, how you feel today? ___

JOURNAL OF HOW I FELT TODAY AND WHAT I ACCOMPLISHED

Be sure your supplements include all of those minerals and vitamins.

DAY 83

Cakes, pies, cookies, etc., are very difficult for me to limit in my diet. I have found it helpful to allow one of these "sweets" one time a week, usually on the weekend.

CHOCOLATE: Allow 1 small serving every 3 days. Note the amount eaten. ____

CARBONATED BEVERAGES: Allow 1 can every 3 days. Drink less if possible. Enter amount consumed. ____

COFFEE: Allow no more than 1 cup today. Number of cups consumed today. ____

ALCOHOL: Allow no more than 1 drink every 3 days. Write number consumed. ____

CIGARETTES: Try to smoke 2 or fewer cigarettes. Write number smoked today. ____

REFINED SUGARS: Limit sugars to 2 servings a week and breads and pastas to 3 servings. Enter number of servings consumed. ____

WATER: Drink 8 glasses of water. Note number of glasses. ____

Replace red meat with one of the following.

beans	____	tofu	____	eggs	____	sprouts	____
almonds	____	TVP	____	cashews	____	chicken	____
turkey	____	lobster	____	salmon	____	tuna	____

EXERCISE: Walk briskly for 35 minutes without stopping. Check here when finished. ____

STRETCHING: Do exercise plan #1. Check here when finished. ____

SLEEP: Continue with ideas from back of workbook.

SUPPLEMENTS: Check here after taking your supplements. ____

ON A SCALE OF 1-10, with 1 indicating the least intensity, how you feel today? ____

JOURNAL OF HOW I FELT TODAY AND WHAT I ACCOMPLISHED

I look forward to a "sweet" treat on the weekend, although I can tell the ill effects it has on my body almost immediately.

DAY 84

According to a number of studies, the average American diet includes over 140 pounds of added sugar per year, which accounts for 18 percent of the average American's caloric intake.

CHOCOLATE: Allow 1 small serving every 3 days. Note the amount eaten. ___

CARBONATED BEVERAGES: Allow 1 can every 3 days. Drink less if possible.

Enter amount consumed. ___

COFFEE: Allow no more than 1 cup today. Number of cups consumed today. ___

ALCOHOL: Allow no more than 1 drink every 3 days. Write number consumed. ___

CIGARETTES: Try to smoke 2 or fewer cigarettes. Write number smoked today. ___

REFINED SUGARS: Limit sugars to 2 servings a week and breads and pastas to 3 servings.

Enter number of servings consumed. ___

WATER: Drink 8 glasses of water. Note number of glasses. ___

Replace red meat with one of the following.

beans	___	tofu	___	eggs	___	sprouts	___
almonds	___	TVP	___	cashews	___	chicken	___
turkey	___	lobster	___	salmon	___	tuna	___

EXERCISE: Walk briskly for 40 minutes without stopping. Check here when finished. ___

STRETCHING: Do exercise plan #1. Check here when finished. ___

SLEEP: Continue with ideas from back of workbook.

SUPPLEMENTS: Check here after taking your supplements. ___

ON A SCALE OF 1-10, with 1 indicating the least intensity, how you feel today? ___

JOURNAL OF HOW I FELT TODAY AND WHAT I ACCOMPLISHED

Added sugar can make our diets a complete disaster. Refined sugar actually helps to break down our immune system, which could make us more susceptible to immune problems.

DAY 85

The various pieces of information contained in this book are "tools" to help you feel good again. You can feel good again, but it's up to you to make the necessary changes to recover.

CHOCOLATE: Allow 1 small serving every 3 days. Note the amount eaten. ___

CARBONATED BEVERAGES: Allow 1 can every 3 days. Drink less if possible.
Enter amount consumed. ___

COFFEE: Allow no more than 1 cup today. Number of cups consumed today. ___

ALCOHOL: Allow no more than 1 drink every 3 days. Write number consumed. ___

CIGARETTES: Try to smoke 2 or fewer cigarettes. Write number smoked today. ___

REFINED SUGARS: Limit sugars to 2 servings a week and breads and pastas to 3 servings.
Enter number of servings consumed. ___

WATER: Drink 8 glasses of water. Note number of glasses. ___

Replace red meat with one of the following.

beans	___	tofu	___	eggs	___	sprouts	___
almonds	___	TVP	___	cashews	___	chicken	___
turkey	___	lobster	___	salmon	___	tuna	___

EXERCISE: Walk briskly for 40 minutes without stopping. Check here when finished. ___

STRETCHING: Do exercise plan #2. Check here when finished. ___

SLEEP: Continue with ideas from back of workbook.

SUPPLEMENTS: Check here after taking your supplements. ___

ON A SCALE OF 1-10, with 1 indicating the least intensity, how you feel today? ___

JOURNAL OF HOW I FELT TODAY AND WHAT I ACCOMPLISHED

Many times we rely completely on pills or doctors to make us feel better. With FMS it takes longer since it takes more time for our bodies to heal.

DAY 86

Part of my maintenance for keeping well has included regular chiropractic adjustments. It has been interesting to feel the differences in my body from when I felt bad compared to now. The adjustments I now need are generally due to back strain from gardening.

CHOCOLATE: Allow 1 small serving every 3 days. Note the amount eaten. ___

CARBONATED BEVERAGES: Allow 1 can every 3 days. Drink less if possible.
Enter amount consumed. ___

COFFEE: Allow no more than 1 cup today. Number of cups consumed today. ___

ALCOHOL: Allow no more than 1 drink every 3 days. Write number consumed. ___

CIGARETTES: Try to smoke 2 or fewer cigarettes. Write number smoked today. ___

REFINED SUGARS: Limit sugars to 2 servings a week and breads and pastas to 3 servings.
Enter number of servings consumed. ___

WATER: Drink 8 glasses of water. Note number of glasses. ___

Replace red meat with one of the following.

beans	___	tofu	___	eggs	___	sprouts	___
almonds	___	TVP	___	cashews	___	chicken	___
turkey	___	lobster	___	salmon	___	tuna	___

EXERCISE: Walk briskly for 40 minutes without stopping. Check here when finished. ___

STRETCHING: Do exercise plan #3. Check here when finished. ___

SLEEP: Continue with ideas from back of workbook.

SUPPLEMENTS: Check here after taking your supplements. ___

ON A SCALE OF 1-10, with 1 indicating the least intensity, how you feel today? ___

JOURNAL OF HOW I FELT TODAY AND WHAT I ACCOMPLISHED

It is important to remember once we get better, we are just like everyone else. We still may have physical problems from time to time, although the difference is our physical problems are no longer "chronic" problems.

DAY 87

Something that has been brought to my attention by the medical profession is the fact that those of us with FMS seem to continually have a negative attitude.

CHOCOLATE: Allow 1 small serving every 3 days. Note the amount eaten. ___
CARBONATED BEVERAGES: Allow 1 can every 3 days. Drink less if possible.
Enter amount consumed. ___
COFFEE: Allow no more than 1 cup today. Number of cups consumed today. ___
ALCOHOL: Allow no more than 1 drink every 3 days. Write number consumed. ___
CIGARETTES: Try to smoke 2 or fewer cigarettes. Write number smoked today. ___
REFINED SUGARS: Limit sugars to 2 servings a week and breads and pastas to 3 servings.
Enter number of servings consumed. ___
WATER: Drink 8 glasses of water. Note number of glasses. ___

Replace red meat with one of the following.

beans	___	tofu	___	eggs	___	sprouts	___
almonds	___	TVP	___	cashews	___	chicken	___
turkey	___	lobster	___	salmon	___	tuna	___

EXERCISE: Walk briskly for 40 minutes without stopping. Check here when finished. ___
STRETCHING: Do exercise plan #1. Check here when finished. ___
SLEEP: Continue with ideas from back of workbook.
SUPPLEMENTS: Check here after taking your supplements. ___
ON A SCALE OF 1-10, with 1 indicating the least intensity, how you feel today? ___

JOURNAL OF HOW I FELT TODAY AND WHAT I ACCOMPLISHED

Our attitude is one of the major hurdles for us to overcome to get well! Try not to think "coping" or "poor me," but begin to think how good it will be to be well again!

DAY 88

It is still important for me to take about 20 minutes every day to sit or lie in a comfortable place and just be still. I try not to think of anything, just be.

CHOCOLATE: Allow 1 small serving every 3 days. Note the amount eaten.   ___

CARBONATED BEVERAGES: Allow 1 can every 3 days. Drink less if possible.
Enter amount consumed.   ___

COFFEE: Allow no more than 1 cup today. Number of cups consumed today.   ___

ALCOHOL: Allow no more than 1 drink every 3 days. Write number consumed.   ___

CIGARETTES: Try to smoke 2 or fewer cigarettes. Write number smoked today.   ___

REFINED SUGARS: Limit sugars to 2 servings a week and breads and pastas to 3 servings.
Enter number of servings consumed.   ___

WATER: Drink 8 glasses of water. Note number of glasses.   ___

Replace red meat with one of the following.

beans	___	tofu	___	eggs	___	sprouts	___
almonds	___	TVP	___	cashews	___	chicken	___
turkey	___	lobster	___	salmon	___	tuna	___

EXERCISE: Walk briskly for 40 minutes without stopping. Check here when finished.   ___

STRETCHING: Do exercise plan #2. Check here when finished.   ___

SLEEP: Continue with ideas from back of workbook.

SUPPLEMENTS: Check here after taking your supplements.   ___

ON A SCALE OF 1-10, with 1 indicating the least intensity, how you feel today?   ___

JOURNAL OF HOW I FELT TODAY AND WHAT I ACCOMPLISHED

After a short period of time it becomes very easy. I especially like to do this during the day when things are very quiet.

DAY 89

Thinking positively is not so difficult to do once we accept the basic premise that there is a greater force which has built this beautiful home for us.

CHOCOLATE: Allow 1 small serving every 3 days. Note the amount eaten.

CARBONATED BEVERAGES: Allow 1 can every 3 days. Drink less if possible. Enter amount consumed. ___

COFFEE: Allow no more than 1 cup today. Number of cups consumed today. ___

ALCOHOL: Allow no more than 1 drink every 3 days. Write number consumed. ___

CIGARETTES: Try to smoke 2 or fewer cigarettes. Write number smoked today. ___

REFINED SUGARS: Limit sugars to 2 servings a week and breads and pastas to 3 servings. Enter number of servings consumed.

WATER: Drink 8 glasses of water. Note number of glasses. ___

Replace red meat with one of the following.

beans	___	tofu	___	eggs	___	sprouts	___
almonds	___	TVP	___	cashews	___	chicken	___
turkey	___	lobster	___	salmon	___	tuna	___

EXERCISE: Walk briskly for 40 minutes without stopping. Check here when finished. ___

STRETCHING: Do exercise plan #3. Check here when finished. ___

SLEEP: Continue with ideas from back of workbook.

SUPPLEMENTS: Check here after taking your supplements.

ON A SCALE OF 1-10, with 1 indicating the least intensity, how you feel today? ___

JOURNAL OF HOW I FELT TODAY AND WHAT I ACCOMPLISHED

I'm not thinking about a man made structure. Think about birds, plants and the earth before we humans decided to change the structure of it. Everything in life is as it should be, and we should be careful about how we change it.

DAY 90

Illness may be our body's way of telling us some changes in our eating habits and lifestyle are due.

CHOCOLATE: Allow 1 small serving every 3 days. Note the amount eaten.   ___
CARBONATED BEVERAGES: Allow 1 can every 3 days. Drink less if possible.
Enter amount consumed.   ___
COFFEE: Allow no more than 1 cup today. Number of cups consumed today.   ___
ALCOHOL: Allow no more than 1 drink every 3 days. Write number consumed.   ___
CIGARETTES: Try to smoke 2 or fewer cigarettes. Write number smoked today.   ___
REFINED SUGARS: Limit sugars to 2 servings a week and breads and pastas to 3 servings.
Enter number of servings consumed.   ___
WATER: Drink 8 glasses of water. Note number of glasses.   ___

Replace red meat with one of the following.

beans	___	tofu	___	eggs	___	sprouts	___
almonds	___	TVP	___	cashews	___	chicken	___
turkey	___	lobster	___	salmon	___	tuna	___

EXERCISE: Walk briskly for 40 minutes without stopping. Check here when finished.   ___
STRETCHING: Do exercise plan #1. Check here when finished.   ___
SLEEP: Continue with ideas from back of workbook.
SUPPLEMENTS: Check here after taking your supplements.   ___
ON A SCALE OF 1-10, with 1 indicating the least intensity, how you feel today?   ___

JOURNAL OF HOW I FELT TODAY AND WHAT I ACCOMPLISHED

This is our opportunity to get in alignment with our creator and help improve the gift so generously given us, our bodies.

Congratulations!

You've made it through another month! You have one more month left to finish the book! Keep up the good work.

If family and friends are not as supportive as you would like, remember that it can be difficult for them too. Neverending caregiving and sympathy is hard to maintain. In their own way, they may feel as hopeless about your situation as you did before you started with this program. Talk to them about your areas of improvement. Focus on the positive, and it will help them and, guess what? It will help you, too! (The above was written by my husband, Karl, to help us know how our loved ones may feel.)

It's Not the Destination . . .
It's the Journey

It's not where you end up that means as much
As the road that you travel along.
And it's not the result that counts as such
As the way that makes you strong.
Since, it's not the destination . . .
It's the journey.

It's not meeting your aim that matters as much
As the course that you take to get there.
And it's not reaching the goal but who you touch
As the path's deeper meaning you share.
Because, it's not the destination . . .
It's the journey.

It's not realizing the objective that you meet
As the trail's challenge that you weather.
And it's not making the finish but who you greet
As on the highway you walk together.
You see, it's not the destination . . .
It's the journey.

Arlene Alpert

Health Evaluation Form

Refer back to this page only one time per month; after you have filled out the HEF for the next month.

Indicate in the column next to the symptoms which of the following conditions apply to you in terms of frequency and/or intensity of symptoms using the numbers 1-10: 1 being the least amount of intensity and 10 being the greatest. After filling it out, refer to the HEF form filled out in the front section of the workbook to compare the differences.

Low energy/Often feel tired			Light sleep/aware of surroundings	
Skin problems–dry, itchy, acne			Cold hands and feet	
Headaches/migraines			Shortness of breath	
Aching joints			Often feel bloated	
Muscle cramps			Bowel gas	
Menstrual cramps/moody/PMS			Heartburn/indigestion	
Cuts and bruises heal slowly			Constipation/diarrhea	
Poor concentration			Weak fingernails/Unhealthy hair	
Difficulty handling stress			Poor muscle tone	
Strong desire for sweets/salts			Water retention	
High/low blood pressure			Cellulite	
Frequently take pain killers			Allergies/Hayfever	
Moods of depression			Poor night vision	
Difficulty getting up in morning			Varicose veins	
Difficulty falling asleep			Hemorrhoids	

How many glasses of water do you drink each day? ____

How many cups of coffee do you drink each day? ____

How many times do you drink alcohol each day? ____

How many cans of pop do you drink each day? ____

How many times do you eat chocolate each day? ____

How many times do you eat red meat each day? ____

How much weight have you gained in the past year? ____

DAY 91

Know in your heart that you can feel well and energetic again. Keep that thought in your mind always, even on those bad days. Then thank your body for responding to the help you are giving it.

CHOCOLATE: Allow 1 small serving every 3 days. Note the amount eaten.   ___

CARBONATED BEVERAGES: Allow 1 can every 3 days. Drink less if possible.
Enter amount consumed.   ___

COFFEE: Allow no more than 1 cup today. Number of cups consumed today.   ___

ALCOHOL: Allow no more than 1 drink every 3 days. Write number consumed.   ___

CIGARETTES: Try to smoke 2 or fewer cigarettes. Write number smoked today.   ___

REFINED SUGARS: Limit sugars to 2 servings a week and breads and pastas to 3 servings.
Enter number of servings consumed.   ___

WATER: Drink 8 glasses of water. Note number of glasses.   ___

If you aren't having red meat today, replace protein with one of the following.

beans	___	tofu	___	eggs	___	sprouts	___
almonds	___	TVP	___	cashews	___	chicken	___
turkey	___	lobster	___	salmon	___	tuna	___

EXERCISE: Walk briskly for 40 minutes without stopping. Check here when finished.   ___

STRETCHING: Do exercise plan #2. Check here when finished.   ___

SLEEP: Continue with ideas from back of workbook.

SUPPLEMENTS: Check here after taking your supplements.   ___

ON A SCALE OF 1-10, with 1 indicating the least intensity, how you feel today?   ___

JOURNAL OF HOW I FELT TODAY AND WHAT I ACCOMPLISHED

You can feel great again; I'm living proof. In the next few days, I will give you some examples of how far I've come.

DAY 92

In 1982, while living in Des Moines, Iowa, I was in and out of doctor's offices often. The pain in my abdomen had become so severe that I felt as if a knife was in there at all times, twisting around with every move.

CHOCOLATE: Allow 1 small serving every 3 days. Note the amount eaten. ⸺

CARBONATED BEVERAGES: Allow 1 can every 3 days. Drink less if possible.

Enter amount consumed. ⸺

COFFEE: Allow no more than 1 cup today. Number of cups consumed today. ⸺

ALCOHOL: Allow no more than 1 drink every 3 days. Write number consumed. ⸺

CIGARETTES: Try to smoke 2 or fewer cigarettes. Write number smoked today. ⸺

REFINED SUGARS: Limit sugars to 2 servings a week and breads and pastas to 3 servings.

Enter number of servings consumed. ⸺

WATER: Drink 8 glasses of water. Note number of glasses. ⸺

If you aren't having red meat today, replace protein with one of the following.

beans	⸺	tofu	⸺	eggs	⸺	sprouts	⸺
almonds	⸺	TVP	⸺	cashews	⸺	chicken	⸺
turkey	⸺	lobster	⸺	salmon	⸺	tuna	⸺

EXERCISE: Walk briskly for 40 minutes without stopping. Check here when finished. ⸺

STRETCHING: Do exercise plan #3. Check here when finished. ⸺

SLEEP: Continue with ideas from back of workbook.

SUPPLEMENTS: Check here after taking your supplements. ⸺

ON A SCALE OF 1-10, with 1 indicating the least intensity, how you feel today? ⸺

JOURNAL OF HOW I FELT TODAY AND WHAT I ACCOMPLISHED

During that time I became so weak that I would have to rest after walking across a four lane highway.

DAY 93

During this same period, pain and weakness became my personal bodyguard. I was now unable to work, so I would spend the entire afternoon planning and making the evening meal so it would be ready for my husband and our son by early evening.

CHOCOLATE: Allow 1 small serving every 3 days. Note the amount eaten. ___

CARBONATED BEVERAGES: Allow 1 can every 3 days. Drink less if possible. Enter amount consumed. ___

COFFEE: Allow no more than 1 cup today. Number of cups consumed today. ___

ALCOHOL: Allow no more than 1 drink every 3 days. Write number consumed. ___

CIGARETTES: Try to smoke 2 or fewer cigarettes. Write number smoked today. ___

REFINED SUGARS: Limit sugars to 2 servings a week and breads and pastas to 3 servings. Enter number of servings consumed. ___

WATER: Drink 8 glasses of water. Note number of glasses. ___

If you aren't having red meat today, replace protein with one of the following.

beans	___	tofu	___	eggs	___	sprouts	___
almonds	___	TVP	___	cashews	___	chicken	___
turkey	___	lobster	___	salmon	___	tuna	___

EXERCISE: Walk briskly for 40 minutes without stopping. Check here when finished. ___

STRETCHING: Do exercise plan #1. Check here when finished. ___

SLEEP: Continue with ideas from back of workbook.

SUPPLEMENTS: Check here after taking your supplements. ___

ON A SCALE OF 1-10, with 1 indicating the least intensity, how you feel today? ___

JOURNAL OF HOW I FELT TODAY AND WHAT I ACCOMPLISHED

I would do one segment of the meal at a time, then go into the living room and lay down until I could get the strength to do another segment. (Does this sound familiar?)

DAY 94

In 1992, six years after being diagnosed and told to "live with it," memory lapses became an every hour occurrence. Many times I would forget the topic while in the midst of a conversation.

CHOCOLATE: Allow 1 small serving every 3 days. Note the amount eaten. ___

CARBONATED BEVERAGES: Allow 1 can every 3 days. Drink less if possible. Enter amount consumed. ___

COFFEE: Allow no more than 1 cup today. Number of cups consumed today. ___

ALCOHOL: Allow no more than 1 drink every 3 days. Write number consumed. ___

CIGARETTES: Try to smoke 2 or fewer cigarettes. Write number smoked today. ___

REFINED SUGARS: Limit sugars to 2 servings a week and breads and pastas to 3 servings. Enter number of servings consumed. ___

WATER: Drink 8 glasses of water. Note number of glasses. ___

If you aren't having red meat today, replace protein with one of the following.

beans ___	tofu ___	eggs ___	sprouts ___
almonds ___	TVP ___	cashews ___	chicken ___
turkey ___	lobster ___	salmon ___	tuna ___

EXERCISE: Walk briskly for 40 minutes without stopping. Check here when finished. ___

STRETCHING: Do exercise plan #2. Check here when finished. ___

SLEEP: Continue with ideas from back of workbook.

SUPPLEMENTS: Check here after taking your supplements. ___

ON A SCALE OF 1-10, with 1 indicating the least intensity, how you feel today? ___

JOURNAL OF HOW I FELT TODAY AND WHAT I ACCOMPLISHED

Since I was teaching at that time, the students would get a number of breaks to allow me to remember what I had been teaching. I'll bet that I was one of the most popular teachers on campus!

DAY 95

In 1992, six years after being diagnosed and told to "live with it," memory lapses became an every hour occurrence. Many times I would forget the topic while in the midst of a conversation.

CHOCOLATE: Allow 1 small serving every 3 days. Note the amount eaten.

CARBONATED BEVERAGES: Allow 1 can every 3 days. Drink less if possible. Enter amount consumed. ___

COFFEE: Allow no more than 1 cup today. Number of cups consumed today. ___

ALCOHOL: Allow no more than 1 drink every 3 days. Write number consumed. ___

CIGARETTES: Try to smoke 2 or fewer cigarettes. Write number smoked today. ___

REFINED SUGARS: Limit sugars to 2 servings a week and breads and pastas to 3 servings. Enter number of servings consumed.

WATER: Drink 8 glasses of water. Note number of glasses. ___

If you aren't having red meat today, replace protein with one of the following.

beans	___	tofu	___	eggs	___	sprouts	___
almonds	___	TVP	___	cashews	___	chicken	___
turkey	___	lobster	___	salmon	___	tuna	___

EXERCISE: Walk briskly for 40 minutes without stopping. Check here when finished. ___

STRETCHING: Do exercise plan #3. Check here when finished. ___

SLEEP: Continue with ideas from back of workbook.

SUPPLEMENTS: Check here after taking your supplements. ___

ON A SCALE OF 1-10, with 1 indicating the least intensity, how you feel today? ___

JOURNAL OF HOW I FELT TODAY AND WHAT I ACCOMPLISHED

Have you ever known anyone who has beaten cancer with a negative outlook on life? Think about it: it doesn't generally happen that way.

DAY 96

In addition to feeling better, one of the benefits I have discovered from using this program is weight loss! Once my body was able to dunction properly, and was getting the proper nutrients, my metabolism increased and the weight decreased.

CHOCOLATE: Allow 1 small serving every 3 days. Note the amount eaten. ⎯

CARBONATED BEVERAGES: Allow 1 can every 3 days. Drink less if possible.
Enter amount consumed. ⎯

COFFEE: Allow no more than 1 cup today. Number of cups consumed today. ⎯

ALCOHOL: Allow no more than 1 drink every 3 days. Write number consumed. ⎯

CIGARETTES: Try to smoke 2 or fewer cigarettes. Write number smoked today. ⎯

REFINED SUGARS: Limit sugars to 2 servings a week and breads and pastas to 3 servings.
Enter number of servings consumed. ⎯

WATER: Drink 8 glasses of water. Note number of glasses. ⎯

If you aren't having red meat today, replace protein with one of the following.

beans	⎯	tofu	⎯	eggs	⎯	sprouts	⎯
almonds	⎯	TVP	⎯	cashews	⎯	chicken	⎯
turkey	⎯	lobster	⎯	salmon	⎯	tuna	⎯

EXERCISE: Walk briskly for 40 minutes without stopping. Check here when finished. ⎯

STRETCHING: Do exercise plan #3. Check here when finished. ⎯

SLEEP: Continue with ideas from back of workbook.

SUPPLEMENTS: Check here after taking your supplements. ⎯

ON A SCALE OF 1-10, with 1 indicating the least intensity, how you feel today? ⎯

JOURNAL OF HOW I FELT TODAY AND WHAT I ACCOMPLISHED

You can do it. You have gotten this far, keep up the good work. Imagine yourself doing all the things you love doing and keep that thought in your mind as your goal.

DAY 97

You have almost made it through this program! Congratulations! We will be making a few more changes at day 100. Remember, the first four items in the list below must be completely deleted from our diets to feel completely well again.

CHOCOLATE: Allow 1 small serving every 3 days. Note the amount eaten. ___

CARBONATED BEVERAGES: Allow 1 can every 3 days. Drink less if possible. Enter amount consumed. ___

COFFEE: Allow no more than 1 cup today. Number of cups consumed today. ___

ALCOHOL: Allow no more than 1 drink every 3 days. Write number consumed. ___

CIGARETTES: Try to smoke 2 or fewer cigarettes. Write number smoked today. ___

REFINED SUGARS: Limit sugars to 2 servings a week and breads and pastas to 3 servings. Enter number of servings consumed. ___

WATER: Drink 8 glasses of water. Note number of glasses. ___

If you aren't having red meat today, replace protein with one of the following.

beans	___	tofu	___	eggs	___	sprouts	___
almonds	___	TVP	___	cashews	___	chicken	___
turkey	___	lobster	___	salmon	___	tuna	___

EXERCISE: Walk briskly for 40 minutes without stopping. Check here when finished. ___

STRETCHING: Do exercise plan #3. Check here when finished. ___

SLEEP: Continue with ideas from back of workbook.

SUPPLEMENTS: Check here after taking your supplements. ___

ON A SCALE OF 1-10, with 1 indicating the least intensity, how you feel today? ___

JOURNAL OF HOW I FELT TODAY AND WHAT I ACCOMPLISHED

You are almost through the first half of the program. You have made it through the worst times in terms of beginning to make the necessary changes. You're doing great, keep up the good work!

DAY 98

Getting and keeping a positive attitude can be accomplished in a number of ways. Each person must find a way that works best for them. An important factor to remember is to tell yourself you will start looking at negatives in a positive manner.

CHOCOLATE: Allow 1 small serving every 3 days. Note the amount eaten.   ___

CARBONATED BEVERAGES: Allow 1 can every 3 days. Drink less if possible.

Enter amount consumed.   ___

COFFEE: Allow no more than 1 cup today. Number of cups consumed today.   ___

ALCOHOL: Allow no more than 1 drink every 3 days. Write number consumed.   ___

CIGARETTES: Try to smoke 2 or fewer cigarettes. Write number smoked today.   ___

REFINED SUGARS: Limit sugars to 2 servings a week and breads and pastas to 3 servings.

Enter number of servings consumed.   ___

WATER: Drink 8 glasses of water. Note number of glasses.   ___

If you aren't having red meat today, replace protein with one of the following.

beans	___	tofu	___	eggs	___	sprouts	___
almonds	___	TVP	___	cashews	___	chicken	___
turkey	___	lobster	___	salmon	___	tuna	___

EXERCISE: Walk briskly for 40 minutes without stopping. Check here when finished.   ___

STRETCHING: Do exercise plan #1. Check here when finished.   ___

SLEEP: Continue with ideas from back of workbook.

SUPPLEMENTS: Check here after taking your supplements.   ___

ON A SCALE OF 1-10, with 1 indicating the least intensity, how you feel today?   ___

JOURNAL OF HOW I FELT TODAY AND WHAT I ACCOMPLISHED

For instance, today challenge yourself. For just two hours allow no negative thoughts into your mind. Each time you start thinking in a negative manner, replace that thought with a positive one.

DAY 99

How did you do yesterday with the positive thinking? I found it to be somewhat hard at first, but believe me, it gets easier!

CHOCOLATE: Allow 1 small serving every 3 days. Note the amount eaten. ___

CARBONATED BEVERAGES: Allow 1 can every 3 days. Drink less if possible.
Enter amount consumed. ___

COFFEE: Allow no more than 1 cup today. Number of cups consumed today. ___

ALCOHOL: Allow no more than 1 drink every 3 days. Write number consumed. ___

CIGARETTES: Try to smoke 2 or fewer cigarettes. Write number smoked today. ___

REFINED SUGARS: Limit sugars to 2 servings a week and breads and pastas to 3 servings.
Enter number of servings consumed. ___

WATER: Drink 8 glasses of water. Note number of glasses. ___

If you aren't having red meat today, replace protein with one of the following.

beans	___	tofu	___	eggs	___	sprouts	___
almonds	___	TVP	___	cashews	___	chicken	___
turkey	___	lobster	___	salmon	___	tuna	___

EXERCISE: Walk briskly for 40 minutes without stopping. Check here when finished. ___

STRETCHING: Do exercise plan #2. Check here when finished. ___

SLEEP: Continue with ideas from back of workbook.

SUPPLEMENTS: Check here after taking your supplements. ___

ON A SCALE OF 1-10, with 1 indicating the least intensity, how you feel today? ___

JOURNAL OF HOW I FELT TODAY AND WHAT I ACCOMPLISHED

Today continue to turn negative thoughts into positive ones for two hours at a time. It may take a few days to become aware of thinking negatively, but before long you will remind yourself each time a negative thought comes to mind.

DAY 100

Yes! You've made it to the century point in your process of getting better! Remember that I told you it would take 4-6 months to see many benefits. You are almost to the end of the fourth month.

CHOCOLATE: Allow 1 small serving every 3 days. Note the amount eaten. ___

CARBONATED BEVERAGES: Allow 1 can every 3 days. Drink less if possible. Enter amount consumed. ___

COFFEE: Allow no more than 1 cup today. Number of cups consumed today. ___

ALCOHOL: Allow no more than 1 drink every 3 days. Write number consumed. ___

CIGARETTES: Try to smoke 2 or fewer cigarettes. Write number smoked today. ___

REFINED SUGARS: Limit sugars to 2 servings a week and breads and pastas to 3 servings. Enter number of servings consumed. ___

WATER: Drink 8 glasses of water. Note number of glasses. ___

If you aren't having red meat today, replace protein with one of the following.

beans ___	tofu ___	eggs ___	sprouts ___
almonds ___	TVP ___	cashews ___	chicken ___
turkey ___	lobster ___	salmon ___	tuna ___

EXERCISE: Walk briskly for 40 minutes without stopping. Check here when finished. ___

STRETCHING: Do exercise plan #3. Check here when finished. ___

SLEEP: Continue with ideas from back of workbook.

SUPPLEMENTS: Check here after taking your supplements. ___

ON A SCALE OF 1-10, with 1 indicating the least intensity, how you feel today? ___

JOURNAL OF HOW I FELT TODAY AND WHAT I ACCOMPLISHED

You may still have some bad days, but you should start noticing the bad days aren't as bad as before. That is where the journal comes in. You can look back at each day to remind yourself of where you've come from.

DAY 101

We will make some changes today. Some of these should be a little easier than at the beginning. Remember that we are working on lifestyle changes, not changes for today.

CHOCOLATE: Allow 1 small serving per week. Note the amount eaten. ___
CARBONATED BEVERAGES: Allow 1 can per week. Enter amount consumed. ___
COFFEE: Allow 1 cup every other day. Number of cups consumed today. ___
ALCOHOL: Allow 1 drink every week. Write number consumed. ___
CIGARETTES: Allow 1 cigarette. This is your treat, so don't smoke it until you have to. ___
REFINED SUGARS: Limit sugars to 2 servings a week. Enter number consumed. ___
WATER: Drink 8 glasses of water. Note number of glasses. ___

If you aren't having red meat today, replace protein with one of the following.

beans	___	tofu	___	eggs	___	sprouts	___
almonds	___	TVP	___	cashews	___	chicken	___
turkey	___	lobster	___	salmon	___	tuna	___

EXERCISE: Walk briskly for 40 minutes without stopping. Check here when finished. ___
STRETCHING: Do exercise plan #3. Check here when finished. ___
SLEEP: Continue with ideas from back of workbook.
SUPPLEMENTS: Check here after taking your supplements. ___
ON A SCALE OF 1-10, with 1 indicating the least intensity, how you feel today? ___

JOURNAL OF HOW I FELT TODAY AND WHAT I ACCOMPLISHED

At this time if you find it easier to cut any of the top four items out completely, go ahead and do it.

DAY 102

Another way to start looking at life more positively is to begin taking some quiet time for about 15 minutes each day. This also helps revitalize the body and spirit.

CHOCOLATE: Allow 1 small serving per week. Note the amount eaten. ____

CARBONATED BEVERAGES: Allow 1 can per week. Enter amount consumed. ____

COFFEE: Allow 1 cup every other day. Keep up the good work!
Number of cups consumed today. ____

ALCOHOL: Allow 1 drink every week. Write number consumed. ____

CIGARETTES: Allow 1 cigarette. This is your treat, so don't smoke it until you have to. ____

REFINED SUGARS: Limit sugars to 2 servings a week. Enter number consumed. ____

WATER: Drink 8 glasses of water. Note number of glasses. ____

If you aren't having red meat today, replace protein with one of the following.

beans	____	tofu	____	eggs	____	sprouts	____
almonds	____	TVP	____	cashews	____	chicken	____
turkey	____	lobster	____	salmon	____	tuna	____

EXERCISE: Walk briskly for 40 minutes without stopping. Check here when finished. ____

STRETCHING: Do exercise plan #1. Check here when finished. ____

SLEEP: Continue with ideas from back of workbook.

SUPPLEMENTS: Check here after taking your supplements. ____

ON A SCALE OF 1-10, with 1 indicating the least intensity, how you feel today? ____

JOURNAL OF HOW I FELT TODAY AND WHAT I ACCOMPLISHED

In the next few days, we will learn how to quiet our mind and body. Many times in my seminars people will say they can't get their minds to become quiet.

DAY 103

Find a quiet place with no distractions. In warm weather, I find my favorite place is lying on a rug in the grass. If it is in the morning, I let the singing birds provide music. Otherwise, I may turn on a tape with sounds of instruments or nature.

CHOCOLATE: Allow 1 small serving per week. Note the amount eaten.   ___

CARBONATED BEVERAGES: Allow 1 can per week. Enter amount consumed.   ___

COFFEE: Allow 1 cup every other day. Keep up the good work!
Number of cups consumed today.

ALCOHOL: Allow 1 drink every week. Write number consumed.   ___

CIGARETTES: Allow 1 cigarette. This is your treat, so don't smoke it until you have to.   ___

REFINED SUGARS: Limit sugar foods to 2 servings a week. Enter number consumed.   ___

WATER: Drink 8 glasses of water. Note number of glasses.   ___

If you aren't having red meat today, replace protein with one of the following.

beans	___	tofu	___	eggs	___	sprouts	___
almonds	___	TVP	___	cashews	___	chicken	___
turkey	___	lobster	___	salmon	___	tuna	___

EXERCISE: Walk briskly for 40 minutes without stopping. Check here when finished.   ___

STRETCHING: Do exercise plan #1. Check here when finished.   ___

SLEEP: Continue with ideas from back of workbook.

SUPPLEMENTS: Check here after taking your supplements.   ___

ON A SCALE OF 1-10, with 1 indicating the least intensity, how you feel today?   ___

JOURNAL OF HOW I FELT TODAY AND WHAT I ACCOMPLISHED

Lay down with your feet about hip width apart and hands out some from the body with palms facing upwards. Now gently tell your toes to go to sleep, next your ankles, next your legs, then work your way up through the rest of your body (see Day 104 to continue).

DAY 104

Once you get to the face, gently tell all the muscles including the mouth to relax. Now concentrate on a wonderful place you would like to be in. A place that is peaceful and serene, maybe by a waterfall, or in a flower garden, or in a wheat field with the wind blowing through the plants.

CHOCOLATE: Allow 1 small serving per week. Note the amount eaten.   ___

CARBONATED BEVERAGES: Allow 1 can per week. Enter amount consumed.   ___

COFFEE: Allow 1 cup every other day. Keep up the good work!
Number of cups consumed today.   ___

ALCOHOL: Allow 1 drink every week. Write number consumed.   ___

CIGARETTES: Allow 1 cigarette. This is your treat, so don't smoke it until you have to.   ___

REFINED SUGARS: Limit sugar foods to 2 servings a week. Enter number consumed.   ___

WATER: Drink 8 glasses of water. Note number of glasses.   ___

If you aren't having red meat today, replace protein with one of the following.

beans	___	tofu	___	eggs	___	sprouts	___
almonds	___	TVP	___	cashews	___	chicken	___
turkey	___	lobster	___	salmon	___	tuna	___

EXERCISE: Walk briskly for 40 minutes without stopping. Check here when finished.   ___

STRETCHING: Do exercise plan #2. Check here when finished.   ___

SLEEP: Continue with ideas from back of workbook.

SUPPLEMENTS: Check here after taking your supplements.   ___

ON A SCALE OF 1-10, with 1 indicating the least intensity, how you feel today?   ___

JOURNAL OF HOW I FELT TODAY AND WHAT I ACCOMPLISHED

Remind yourself to open your eyes when 15 minutes are up. During this 15 minutes, lay in the peace of the moment. Whenever another thought comes to mind, gently push it out and return to the peaceful setting.

DAY 105

If the relaxing exercise is done on a daily basis, you soon will become more aware of everything around you, including your bodily needs. Your body will begin to let you know when you are doing or eating what you shouldn't.

CHOCOLATE: Allow 1 small serving per week. Note the amount eaten. ___
CARBONATED BEVERAGES: Allow 1 can per week. Enter amount consumed. ___
COFFEE: Allow 1 cup every other day. Keep up the good work!
Number of cups consumed today. ___
ALCOHOL: Allow 1 drink every week. Write number consumed. ___
CIGARETTES: Allow 1 cigarette. This is your treat, so don't smoke it until you have to. ___
REFINED SUGARS: Limit sugar foods to 2 servings a week. Enter number consumed. ___
WATER: Drink 8 glasses of water. Note number of glasses. ___

If you aren't having red meat today, replace protein with one of the following.

beans	___	tofu	___	eggs	___	sprouts	___
almonds	___	TVP	___	cashews	___	chicken	___
turkey	___	lobster	___	salmon	___	tuna	___

EXERCISE: Walk briskly for 40 minutes without stopping. Check here when finished. ___
STRETCHING: Do exercise plan #3. Check here when finished. ___
SLEEP: Continue with ideas from back of workbook.
SUPPLEMENTS: Check here after taking your supplements. ___
ON A SCALE OF 1-10, with 1 indicating the least intensity, how you feel today? ___

JOURNAL OF HOW I FELT TODAY AND WHAT I ACCOMPLISHED

You may also notice you have more patience and are generally more relaxed.

DAY 106

Often sleep aids need to be changed on a regular basis. For instance, if melatonin is taken daily, it may build up in your system to a point that it no longer works as well as it did in the beginning.

CHOCOLATE: Allow 1 small serving per week. Note the amount eaten.   ———

CARBONATED BEVERAGES: Allow 1 can per week. Enter amount consumed.   ———

COFFEE: Allow 1 cup every other day. Keep up the good work!
Number of cups consumed today.   ———

ALCOHOL: Allow 1 drink every week. Write number consumed.   ———

CIGARETTES: Allow 1 cigarette. This is your treat, so don't smoke it until you have to.   ———

REFINED SUGARS: Limit sugar foods to 2 servings a week. Enter number consumed.   ———

WATER: Drink 8 glasses of water. Note number of glasses.   ———

If you aren't having red meat today, replace protein with one of the following.

beans	___	tofu	___	eggs	___	sprouts	___
almonds	___	TVP	___	cashews	___	chicken	___
turkey	___	lobster	___	salmon	___	tuna	___

EXERCISE: Walk briskly for 40 minutes without stopping. Check here when finished.   ___

STRETCHING: Do exercise plan #3. Check here when finished.   ———

SLEEP: Continue with ideas from back of workbook.

SUPPLEMENTS: Check here after taking your supplements.   ———

ON A SCALE OF 1-10, with 1 indicating the least intensity, how you feel today?   ———

JOURNAL OF HOW I FELT TODAY AND WHAT I ACCOMPLISHED

I would take a sleep aid for about 3-4 nights, then use baths and teas 3-4 nights.

DAY 107

Many times health food store remedies for sleep such as passionflower or valerian root are less sedating so there may not be any side effects such as drowsiness in the morning.

CHOCOLATE: Allow 1 small serving per week. Note the amount eaten. ___

CARBONATED BEVERAGES: Allow 1 can per week. Enter amount consumed. ___

COFFEE: Allow 1 cup every other day. Keep up the good work!
Number of cups consumed today. ___

ALCOHOL: Allow 1 drink every week. Write number consumed. ___

CIGARETTES: Allow 1 cigarette. This is your treat, so don't smoke it until you have to. ___

REFINED SUGARS: Limit sugar foods to 2 servings a week. Enter number consumed. ___

WATER: Drink 8 glasses of water. Note number of glasses. ___

If you aren't having red meat today, replace protein with one of the following.

beans	___	tofu	___	eggs	___	sprouts	___
almonds	___	TVP	___	cashews	___	chicken	___
turkey	___	lobster	___	salmon	___	tuna	___

EXERCISE: Walk briskly for 40 minutes without stopping. Check here when finished. ___

STRETCHING: Do exercise plan #3. Check here when finished. ___

SLEEP: Continue with ideas from back of workbook.

SUPPLEMENTS: Check here after taking your supplements. ___

ON A SCALE OF 1-10, with 1 indicating the least intensity, how you feel today? ___

JOURNAL OF HOW I FELT TODAY AND WHAT I ACCOMPLISHED

I enjoy drinking teas more than taking tablets or capsules, since I feel the teas may be absorbed into my system faster which will provide quicker results.

DAY 108

In my garden you'll find mint, chamomile and catnip. Each of these herbs are very easy to grow and when mixed together, make a very nice sleep enhancer as well as a smooth tasting tea.

CHOCOLATE: Allow 1 small serving per week. Note the amount eaten. ___
CARBONATED BEVERAGES: Allow 1 can per week. Enter amount consumed. ___
COFFEE: Allow 1 cup every other day. Keep up the good work!
 Number of cups consumed today. ___
ALCOHOL: Allow 1 drink every week. Write number consumed. ___
CIGARETTES: Allow 1 cigarette. This is your treat, so don't smoke it until you have to. ___
REFINED SUGARS: Limit sugar foods to 2 servings a week. Enter number consumed. ___
WATER: Drink 8 glasses of water. Note number of glasses. ___

If you aren't having red meat today, replace protein with one of the following.

beans	___	tofu	___	eggs	___	sprouts	___
almonds	___	TVP	___	cashews	___	chicken	___
turkey	___	lobster	___	salmon	___	tuna	___

EXERCISE: Walk briskly for 40 minutes without stopping. Check here when finished. ___
STRETCHING: Do exercise plan #2. Check here when finished. ___
SLEEP: Continue with ideas from back of workbook.
SUPPLEMENTS: Check here after taking your supplements. ___
ON A SCALE OF 1-10, with 1 indicating the least intensity, how you feel today? ___

JOURNAL OF HOW I FELT TODAY AND WHAT I ACCOMPLISHED

Pick the flowers of the chamomile and catnip, and put them together with the leaves from the mint in a tea bag. Steep in a cup of boiling water for 5-7 minutes.

DAY 109

I feel it is important to grow a garden, however small it may be. Even if it is in pots, the physical and emotional energy put into that activity is very therapeutic for the mind.

CHOCOLATE: Allow 1 small serving per week. Note the amount eaten. ___

CARBONATED BEVERAGES: Allow 1 can per week. Enter amount consumed. ___

COFFEE: Allow 1 cup every other day. Keep up the good work!
Number of cups consumed today.

ALCOHOL: Allow 1 drink every week. Write number consumed. ___

CIGARETTES: Allow 1 cigarette. This is your treat, so don't smoke it until you have to. ___

REFINED SUGARS: Limit sugar foods to 2 servings a week. Enter number consumed. ___

WATER: Drink 8 glasses of water. Note number of glasses. ___

If you aren't having red meat today, replace protein with one of the following.

beans	___	tofu	___	eggs	___	sprouts	___
almonds	___	TVP	___	cashews	___	chicken	___
turkey	___	lobster	___	salmon	___	tuna	___

EXERCISE: Walk briskly for 40 minutes without stopping. Check here when finished. ___

STRETCHING: Do exercise plan #3. Check here when finished. ___

SLEEP: Continue with ideas from back of workbook.

SUPPLEMENTS: Check here after taking your supplements. ___

ON A SCALE OF 1-10, with 1 indicating the least intensity, how you feel today? ___

JOURNAL OF HOW I FELT TODAY AND WHAT I ACCOMPLISHED

In addition, it can be very economical, considering the money saved in growing your own health aids.

DAY 110

Since it is believed much of the pain of FMS may be caused from a yeast overgrowth in our systems, garlic is another very beneficial herb to keep on hand or in the garden.

CHOCOLATE: Allow 1 small serving per week. Note the amount eaten. ___

CARBONATED BEVERAGES: Allow 1 can per week. Enter amount consumed. ___

COFFEE: Allow 1 cup every other day. Keep up the good work!
Number of cups consumed today. ___

ALCOHOL: Allow 1 drink every week. Write number consumed. ___

CIGARETTES: Allow 1 cigarette. This is your treat, so don't smoke it until you have to. ___

REFINED SUGARS: Limit sugar foods to 2 servings a week. Enter number consumed. ___

WATER: Drink 8 glasses of water. Note number of glasses. ___

If you aren't having red meat today, replace protein with one of the following.

beans ___	tofu ___	eggs ___	sprouts ___
almonds ___	TVP ___	cashews ___	chicken ___
turkey ___	lobster ___	salmon ___	tuna ___

EXERCISE: Walk briskly for 40 minutes without stopping. Check here when finished. ___

STRETCHING: Do exercise plan #1. Check here when finished. ___

SLEEP: Continue with ideas from back of workbook.

SUPPLEMENTS: Check here after taking your supplements. ___

ON A SCALE OF 1-10, with 1 indicating the least intensity, how you feel today? ___

JOURNAL OF HOW I FELT TODAY AND WHAT I ACCOMPLISHED

I first started my garlic patch by buying a garlic bulb, separating the bulbs from the main bulb and planting them about five inches deep. Let at least one of the bulbs bloom and go to seed the first year to keep more plants coming up each year.

DAY 111

Systemic yeast overgrowth many times can cause symptoms of FMS. If your symptoms are caused by a yeast overgrowth, symptoms may be reduced by adding garlic, antifungal medication and live cultured yogurt to your diet, along with adding exercise to your daily routine. Consult with your physician if you think this may be the cause of your symptoms.

CHOCOLATE: Allow 1 small serving per week. Note the amount eaten. ___
CARBONATED BEVERAGES: Allow 1 can per week. Enter amount consumed. ___
COFFEE: Allow 1 cup every other day. Keep up the good work!
Number of cups consumed today.
ALCOHOL: Allow 1 drink every week. Write number consumed. ___
CIGARETTES: Allow 1 cigarette. This is your treat, so don't smoke it until you have to. ___
REFINED SUGARS: Limit sugar foods to 2 servings a week. Enter number consumed. ___
WATER: Drink 8 glasses of water. Note number of glasses. ___

If you aren't having red meat today, replace protein with one of the following.

beans	___	tofu	___	eggs	___	sprouts	___
almonds	___	TVP	___	cashews	___	chicken	___
turkey	___	lobster	___	salmon	___	tuna	___

EXERCISE: Walk briskly for 40 minutes without stopping. Check here when finished. ___
STRETCHING: Do exercise plan #2. Check here when finished. ___
SLEEP: Continue with ideas from back of workbook.
SUPPLEMENTS: Check here after taking your supplements. ___
ON A SCALE OF 1-10, with 1 indicating the least intensity, how you feel today? ___

JOURNAL OF HOW I FELT TODAY AND WHAT I ACCOMPLISHED

I also periodically will drink an immune booster/antitoxin tea to help rid my body of the excess toxins. These teas can be found at your health food stores.

DAY 112

Systemic yeast overgrowth does not show up on typical blood or urine tests. For references on clinics that do specific tests for systemic yeast overgrowth, or books on this topic, refer to the back of the book.

CHOCOLATE: Allow 1 small serving per week. Note the amount eaten. ___
CARBONATED BEVERAGES: Allow 1 can per week. Enter amount consumed. ___
COFFEE: Allow 1 cup every other day. Keep up the good work!
Number of cups consumed today. ___
ALCOHOL: Allow 1 drink every week. Write number consumed. ___
CIGARETTES: Allow 1 cigarette. This is your treat, so don't smoke it until you have to. ___
REFINED SUGARS: Limit sugar foods to 2 servings a week. Enter number consumed. ___
WATER: Drink 8 glasses of water. Note number of glasses. ___

If you aren't having red meat today, replace protein with one of the following.

beans	___	tofu	___	eggs	___	sprouts	___
almonds	___	TVP	___	cashews	___	chicken	___
turkey	___	lobster	___	salmon	___	tuna	___

EXERCISE: Walk briskly for 45 minutes without stopping. Check here when finished. ___
STRETCHING: Do exercise plan #3. Check here when finished. ___
SLEEP: Continue with ideas from back of workbook.
SUPPLEMENTS: Check here after taking your supplements. ___
ON A SCALE OF 1-10, with 1 indicating the least intensity, how you feel today? ___

JOURNAL OF HOW I FELT TODAY AND WHAT I ACCOMPLISHED

Systemic yeast overgrowth can be treated with an antifungal medication, although treatment also includes dietary and other lifestyle changes.

DAY 113

Each time you consume one of the first four items a mild relapse can occur. That is why it is so important to omit those items from your diet.

CHOCOLATE: Allow 1 small serving per week. Note the amount eaten. ___

CARBONATED BEVERAGES: Allow 1 can per week. Enter amount consumed. ___

COFFEE: Allow 1 cup every other day. Keep up the good work! Number of cups consumed today. ___

ALCOHOL: Allow 1 drink every week. Write number consumed. ___

CIGARETTES: Allow 1 cigarette. This is your treat, so don't smoke it until you have to. ___

REFINED SUGARS: Limit sugar foods to 2 servings a week. Enter number consumed. ___

WATER: Drink 8 glasses of water. Note number of glasses. ___

If you aren't having red meat today, replace protein with one of the following.

beans	___	tofu	___	eggs	___	sprouts	___
almonds	___	TVP	___	cashews	___	chicken	___
turkey	___	lobster	___	salmon	___	tuna	___

EXERCISE: Walk briskly for 45 minutes without stopping. Check here when finished. ___

STRETCHING: Do exercise plan #1. Check here when finished. ___

SLEEP: Continue with ideas from back of workbook.

SUPPLEMENTS: Check here after taking your supplements. ___

ON A SCALE OF 1-10, with 1 indicating the least intensity, how you feel today? ___

JOURNAL OF HOW I FELT TODAY AND WHAT I ACCOMPLISHED

The sooner you are able to get those items out of your diet, the sooner you will notice a more dramatic recovery.

DAY 114

A healthy body is one of the greatest gifts we can help ourselves attain. You are well on your way to enjoying this wonderful gift.

CHOCOLATE: Allow 1 small serving per week. Note the amount eaten. ___
CARBONATED BEVERAGES: Allow 1 can per week. Enter amount consumed. ___
COFFEE: Allow 1 cup every other day. Keep up the good work!
Number of cups consumed today. ___
ALCOHOL: Allow 1 drink every week. Write number consumed. ___
CIGARETTES: Allow 1 cigarette. This is your treat, so don't smoke it until you have to. ___
REFINED SUGARS: Limit sugar foods to 2 servings a week. Enter number consumed. ___
WATER: Drink 8 glasses of water. Note number of glasses. ___

If you aren't having red meat today, replace protein with one of the following.

beans ___	tofu ___	eggs ___	sprouts ___
almonds ___	TVP ___	cashews ___	chicken ___
turkey ___	lobster ___	salmon ___	tuna ___

EXERCISE: Walk briskly for 45 minutes without stopping. Check here when finished. ___
STRETCHING: Do exercise plan #2. Check here when finished. ___
SLEEP: Continue with ideas from back of workbook.
SUPPLEMENTS: Check here after taking your supplements. ___
ON A SCALE OF 1-10, with 1 indicating the least intensity, how you feel today? ___

JOURNAL OF HOW I FELT TODAY AND WHAT I ACCOMPLISHED

Your recovery will take time. If a test is taken to see if the symptoms are caused from an overgrowth of yeast, anti-yeast medications can help speed the recovery time.

DAY 115

When you've finished these 4 months in the program, you can continue the program on your own, or purchase the second book of this series.

CHOCOLATE: Allow 1 small serving every other week. Note the amount eaten.

CARBONATED BEVERAGES: Allow 1 can per week. Enter amount consumed. ___

COFFEE: Allow 1 cup every 3rd day, or cut coffee completely from your diet. ___
Number of cups consumed today.

ALCOHOL: Allow 1 drink every other week. Write number consumed. ___

CIGARETTES: Try to quit smoking completely, or limit your donsumption from ___
Day 114. Record number smoked.

REFINED SUGARS: Limit sugar foods to 2 servings a week. Enter number consumed. ___

WATER: Drink 8 glasses of water. Note number of glasses. ___

If you aren't having red meat today, replace protein with one of the following.

beans	___	tofu	___	eggs	___	sprouts	___
almonds	___	TVP	___	cashews	___	chicken	___
turkey	___	lobster	___	salmon	___	tuna	___

EXERCISE: Walk briskly for 45 minutes without stopping. Check here when finished. ___

STRETCHING: Do exercise plan #3. Check here when finished. ___

SLEEP: Continue with ideas from back of workbook.

SUPPLEMENTS: Check here after taking your supplements. ___

ON A SCALE OF 1-10, with 1 indicating the least intensity, how you feel today? ___

JOURNAL OF HOW I FELT TODAY AND WHAT I ACCOMPLISHED

When you finish this book, continue to limit the foods that you have been working to eliminate. It is a life-long process. As time goes on you may be able to "cheat" once in a while. I still "cheat" occasionally, but I enjoy feeling good so much more that those times are getting less frequent.

DAY 116

If you have become tired of trying to feel better, take a day off. That doesn't mean eat, drink or smoke anything you can force into your mouth. If you are frustrated with the amount of time it takes to feel well again, one day off may not be such a bad idea. But only for today!

CHOCOLATE: Allow 1 small serving every other week. Note the amount eaten. ___

CARBONATED BEVERAGES: Allow 1 can per week. Enter amount consumed. ___

COFFEE: Allow 1 cup every 3rd day, or cut coffee completely from your diet.
Number of cups consumed today. ___

ALCOHOL: Allow 1 drink every other week. Write number consumed. ___

CIGARETTES: Try to quit smoking completely, or limit your donsumption from
Day 114. Record number smoked. ___

REFINED SUGARS: Limit sugar foods to 2 servings a week. Enter number consumed. ___

WATER: Drink 8 glasses of water. Note number of glasses. ___

If you aren't having red meat today, replace protein with one of the following.

beans	___	tofu	___	eggs	___	sprouts	___
almonds	___	TVP	___	cashews	___	chicken	___
turkey	___	lobster	___	salmon	___	tuna	___

EXERCISE: Walk briskly for 45 minutes without stopping. Check here when finished. ___

STRETCHING: Do exercise plan #1. Check here when finished. ___

SLEEP: Continue with ideas from back of workbook.

SUPPLEMENTS: Check here after taking your supplements. ___

ON A SCALE OF 1-10, with 1 indicating the least intensity, how you feel today? ___

JOURNAL OF HOW I FELT TODAY AND WHAT I ACCOMPLISHED

If you did "take the day off," you may want to drink a couple of cups of detoxification tea this evening.

DAY 117

As your body becomes healthier, and as you continue to be aware of what to feed it and how to treat it, you may have fewer doctor visits. When my body became healthier, the doctor visits became much less frequent.

CHOCOLATE: Allow 1 small serving every other week. Note the amount eaten. ___
CARBONATED BEVERAGES: Allow 1 can per week. Enter amount consumed. ___
COFFEE: Allow 1 cup every 3rd day, or cut coffee completely from your diet. ___
Number of cups consumed today.
ALCOHOL: Allow 1 drink every other week. Write number consumed. ___
CIGARETTES: Try to quit smoking completely, or limit your donsumption to ___
no more than 1 a day. Record number smoked.
REFINED SUGARS: Limit sugar foods to 2 servings a week. Enter number consumed. ___
WATER: Drink 8 glasses of water. Note number of glasses. ___

If you aren't having red meat today, replace protein with one of the following.

beans	___	tofu	___	eggs	___	sprouts	___
almonds	___	TVP	___	cashews	___	chicken	___
turkey	___	lobster	___	salmon	___	tuna	___

EXERCISE: Walk briskly for 45 minutes without stopping. Check here when finished. ___
STRETCHING: Do exercise plan #2. Check here when finished. ___
SLEEP: Continue with ideas from back of workbook.
SUPPLEMENTS: Check here after taking your supplements.
ON A SCALE OF 1-10, with 1 indicating the least intensity, how you feel today? ___

JOURNAL OF HOW I FELT TODAY AND WHAT I ACCOMPLISHED

Fewer doctor visits translates into fewer dollars spent!

DAY 118

Not only have my doctor visits decreased, my desire to do things that are fun has increased. Imagine what you will do when you are well again, and keep that as your goal.

CHOCOLATE: Allow 1 small serving every other week. Note the amount eaten. ⎯

CARBONATED BEVERAGES: Allow 1 can per week. Enter amount consumed. ⎯

COFFEE: Allow 1 cup every 3rd day, or cut coffee completely from your diet. Number of cups consumed today. ⎯

ALCOHOL: Allow 1 drink every other week. Write number consumed. ⎯

CIGARETTES: Try to quit smoking completely, or limit your consumption to no more than 1 a day. Record number smoked. ⎯

REFINED SUGARS: Limit sugar foods to 2 servings a week. Enter number consumed. ⎯

WATER: Drink 8 glasses of water. Note number of glasses. ⎯

If you aren't having red meat today, replace protein with one of the following.

beans ⎯	tofu ⎯	eggs ⎯	sprouts ⎯
almonds ⎯	TVP ⎯	cashews ⎯	chicken ⎯
turkey ⎯	lobster ⎯	salmon ⎯	tuna ⎯

EXERCISE: Walk briskly for 45 minutes without stopping. Check here when finished. ⎯

STRETCHING: Do exercise plan #3. Check here when finished. ⎯

SLEEP: Continue with ideas from back of workbook.

SUPPLEMENTS: Check here after taking your supplements. ⎯

ON A SCALE OF 1-10, with 1 indicating the least intensity, how you feel today? ⎯

JOURNAL OF HOW I FELT TODAY AND WHAT I ACCOMPLISHED

You've almost made it through 4 months of hard work. By now you should be noticing some improvements in sleep and energy level as well as decreased pain. It is very important to continue on this plan after the book is finished to continue to feel better.

DAY 119

Be sure to go back to the first Health Evaluation Form and compare the results with how you feel today. Then go back and compare your Daily Journal entries to see where the areas of improvement are.

CHOCOLATE: Allow 1 small serving every other week. Note the amount eaten. ___

CARBONATED BEVERAGES: Allow 1 can per week. Enter amount consumed. ___

COFFEE: Allow 1 cup every 3rd day, or cut coffee completely from your diet. Number of cups consumed today.

ALCOHOL: Allow 1 drink every other week. Write number consumed. ___

CIGARETTES: Try to quit smoking completely, or limit your consumption to no more than 1 a day. Record number smoked. ___

REFINED SUGARS: Limit sugar foods to 2 servings a week. Enter number consumed. ___

WATER: Drink 8 glasses of water. Note number of glasses. ___

If you aren't having red meat today, replace protein with one of the following.

beans	___	tofu	___	eggs	___	sprouts	___
almonds	___	TVP	___	cashews	___	chicken	___
turkey	___	lobster	___	salmon	___	tuna	___

EXERCISE: Walk briskly for 45 minutes without stopping. Check here when finished. ___

STRETCHING: Do exercise plan #1. Check here when finished. ___

SLEEP: Continue with ideas from back of workbook.

SUPPLEMENTS: Check here after taking your supplements. ___

ON A SCALE OF 1-10, with 1 indicating the least intensity, how you feel today? ___

JOURNAL OF HOW I FELT TODAY AND WHAT I ACCOMPLISHED

Continue to do your relaxation session 15 minutes each day. It's amazing how much that simple exercise has helped many areas of my health.

DAY 120

It is important to continue the program so your health doesn't slip back. Your body is finally beginning to respond, so it will take time. Continue to take the foods out of your diet that you have been working on. You have made it through part 1! Congratulations, you've done great!!

CHOCOLATE: Allow 1 small serving every other week. Note the amount eaten.   ——

CARBONATED BEVERAGES: Allow 1 can per week. Enter amount consumed.   ——

COFFEE: Allow 1 cup every 3rd day, or cut coffee completely from your diet.
Number of cups consumed today.   ——

ALCOHOL: Allow 1 drink every other week. Write number consumed.

CIGARETTES: Try to quit smoking completely, or limit your consumption to
no more than 1 a day. Record number smoked.   ——

REFINED SUGARS: Limit sugar foods to 2 servings a week. Enter number consumed.   ——

WATER: Drink 8 glasses of water. Note number of glasses.   ——

If you aren't having red meat today, replace protein with one of the following.

beans	——	tofu	——	eggs	——	sprouts	——
almonds	——	TVP	——	cashews	——	chicken	——
turkey	——	lobster	——	salmon	——	tuna	——

EXERCISE: Walk briskly for 45 minutes without stopping. Check here when finished.   ——

STRETCHING: Do exercise plan #2. Check here when finished.   ——

SLEEP: Continue with ideas from back of workbook.

SUPPLEMENTS: Check here after taking your supplements.   ——

ON A SCALE OF 1-10, with 1 indicating the least intensity, how you feel today?   ——

JOURNAL OF HOW I FELT TODAY AND WHAT I ACCOMPLISHED

Congratulations! You've made it through 4 months of *very* hard work. You can feel great again, it's up to you. You're more than half way there. Keep going. Remember that it may take a long time to feel well. You're not alone on this journey. There are many of us out there working on getting better just as you are. Keep up the good work!

Sleep Aids

Herbal Remedies

1. Combination of Mint Leaves and Catnip Flowers

Catnip is considered to be a calmative and mint has qualities that are used to relieve tension, insomnia, nervousness and trembling. Together these herbs make a wonderfully smooth bedtime drink. These herbs are very easy to grow in a garden or in pots which make them an excellent choice. Catnip is also a wonderful immune booster, so it is a very helpful for those who have FMS. To make a tea, pour 1 cup boiling water over mixture of 1 teaspoon catnip flowers and 1 teaspoon mint leaves. Leave to infuse 10 minutes.

2. Chamomile

A warm cup of chamomile tea with a little honey will help to calm the system and promote sleep. Add to mint and catnip leaves in #1 for an even more relaxing drink before going to bed.

3. Lavender

Lavender is a beautiful plant that blooms purple blue flowers. A few have pink or white flowers. It is intensely aromatic. Lavender is a good remedy for headaches, nervous exhaustion and sleeplessness. (of course, none of us exhibit any of those symptoms!)Make a relaxing tea by pouring 1 cup boiling water over 1 teaspoon of fresh flowers. Cover and leave to infuse 10 minutes.

4. Passionflower

Also promotes sleep. This herb is found in health food stores

5. Valerian Root and Lemon Balm

Used to improve deep sleep. Seems to be less sedating than synthetic sleep aids. Can be found in health food stores

6. Melatonin

Helps induce a deep sleep. If used over a period of time, melatonin may not be as effective as if used on an occasional basis. Melatonin actually is not as effective for me as the combination of herbs in #1.

7. Calcium & Magnesium

Increasing daily calcium magnesium intake was very beneficial in helping improve my sleep. I would suggest asking you chiropractor, nutritionist or doctor for help regarding the amount to which you should increase your intake.

Other Sleep Remedies

1. Warm Milk

If you are not sensitive to milk and/or milk products, a cup of warm milk may be all you need. Skim or Acidophilus milk can be used. Heat the milk until it is warm and add 1 tsp. of powdered sugar and 1 tsp. of your favorite flavor. I prefer vanilla. Warming milk is an old time favorite for inducing sleep. As we all know, it works on babies, so why not use it ourselves?

2. Warm Bread

Many times I will include a piece of toast with my cup of warm milk. Warm bread will also help induce sleep.

3. Warm Sage Bath

This is another old remedy I have found to be very beneficial for both sleep and pain control. Fresh sage leaves work best, so summer and fall are good times to get the full benefit from this treatment. In the winter, if I have used all the dried sage from my garden, I will buy a .5 oz bottle of sage. I put the entire content of leaves from the bottle into a muslin tea bag and place it into a quart jar of boiling water. Let it set for 20 minutes. The water should turn medium brown. Pour the tea into the bath and put the tea bag under running water so the water will continue to make tea from the leaves. Soak in the sage bath until the water cools.

4. Reading

Reading may help induce sleep by taking the mind off the feeling that sleeplessness may occur. Find a topic to read which will take you any form stress or feelings of helplessness. For instance I love to read gardening and herbal books. For you, it may be a good love story. It is best not to read while lying in bed, since the bedroom should be thought of as a place to sleep.

5. Massage

Many times I will solicit my daughter or husband to administer wonderful back or foot massage. The massages seem to be even more beneficial after a warm sage bath.

6. Deep Relaxation

Once in bed, many times sleep will come by using the deep relaxation technique. To do this lay on your back and close your eyes. Take at least 3 deep breaths, filling your stomach and chest cavities. Be aware of your breathing, listening to the air moving both in and out as you inhale and exhale. After the deep breathing , begin telling your body to become very heavy and to sleep. I begin with my toes, then my feet, then my ankles, and continue up through my body completing the relaxation with my mouth, tongue, cheeks, eyes, forehead and scalp. Your mouth should be open slightly and you tongue relaxed also. Last, tell your mind to calm and go to sleep. Continue thinking about nothing, gently reminding your mind to stay quiet and relaxed until you find yourself waking up at a later time As a 12 year old on the nights (and they were many!) that I would practice this technique, I was still somewhat aware of my surroundings, but my body felt completely rested the next morning

7. Acupressure

There are a number of different acupressure points that can be used to help induce sleep.

Refer to the chart for the actual pressure points. The series of points around the ribcage and pelvic bones should be done one at a time, moving from one point to the next. Refer to the section on "Acupressure Points" for instructions on how to do the acupressure.

8. Walking

Walking or exercise is a necessary component to getting a good nights sleep since it basically helps the total body become more relaxed and tired. A faster paced walk can actually energize the body, so if you would like to feel energized a brisk walk in the morning will help energize you for the day while helping your body to become tired by the evening hours.

9. Eating

I have found eating too late can affect my sleep drastically. I try to make the evening meal the lightest meal of the day and eat about 3 or more hours before retiring. If I feel hungry just before I go to bed, a banana or other fruit or warm drink will give me a satisfied feeling.

Pain Aids

1. Walking

Walking has been one of the best form to control pain I have found. Many times the pain would be so bad that I could hardly walk. But as I continued to walk the pain would lessen. The walking exercise would also help me achieve a deeper sleep.

2. Gardening

As I continued to feel better, I found gardening seemed to alleviate much of the muscle pain in my back. This is one of the reasons I suggest you start a small garden and grow your own herbs. They are very inexpensive to start and grow, in fact many of the herbal plants I have come from other gardeners. I have found that herbal gardeners are more than happy to share their plants with others. In return I too am sharing any and all the herbs I have with others. Once established, many herbs will come back each year. Herb plants need to be separated every 2-4 years to keep their medicinal potency. The twisting, bending and general movement of gardening helps to stretch muscles and promote better muscle tone while strengthening the body and alleviating pain.

3. Stretching Exercises

The stretching exercises shown in the next section of the book have been my helpers since I was first diagnosed with fibromyalgia in 1986. At the time the doctor suggested I learn exercises in quieting my mind and stretching. I have done them fervently since that time. After a period of time it became easy to know which exercises I needed in that particular day. I still do them at least 4-6 times per week as part of my maintenance program. I include the "quiet time" or deep relaxation for about 10-20 minutes after doing the stretching exercises. Total time for this portion of maintenance is approximately 30 minutes.

4. Sage Bath

This is a great way to help control overall body pain. See instructions on preparing the sage bath in the "Sleep Aids" section.

5, Acupressure

There are many acupressure points to help with muscle tension and pain. Refer to the section on "Acupressure Points" for pain relief.

6. Acupuncture

Acupuncture was very important to help with my symptoms of pain so I could continue making the lifestyle changes necessary to get batter. It is important, though, to find an acupuncturist who has had quite a lot of experience in treating the patient with chronic problems. A needle placed in the wrong median could throw me into a complete relapse.

7. Mental Visualization

This was the first form of pain control I used other than prescription medications, and I found it to be very helpful. To do this sit in a comfortable position and become very relaxed. Focus on the area of intense pain. In you mind see the area becoming warm and pink. (This exercise can be done with the eyes open or closed) Continue to see the are getting warmer and pinker until the pain subsides. For the whole body visualize a pink bubble around you bringing heat and warmth to the entire body. The pink bubble becomes closer and closer to your body and as it is getting closer your body is becoming warmer and pinker. Continue this exercise until the body is very warm and the pain has subsided.

8. Ginger Bath

A ginger bath helps promote circulation. Two ounces of grated ginger are placed in 1 gallon of water and heated but not boiled. Keep the water very hot for 10 minutes. Strain off the ginger. Then add the solution to a hot bath and enjoy!

9. Foods

Sugar and caffeine can help bring on general pain. Take caffeine out of the diet completely and limit sugars to fruits whenever possible. I find munching on any type of melon takes care of my craving for sweets. Grapes are also good for munching.

10 Chiropractic Treatments

Regular chiropractic treatments were necessary for pain control for Kelly and I, although treatments should be very gentle. If too much pressure was put on painful areas I found the treatment had little affect and many times would increase my discomfort. I still get regular chiropractic treatments for "general maintenance".

11. Massage

A good massage therapist can do wonders for the pain and to help promote a good nights sleep.

Note: All of the treatments for pain are only temporary helpers. If diet and lifestyles are not changed, relief from symptoms may be only temporary. We must take responsibility for healing ourselves, and realize treatments and medications should be used as helps to cope with the pain until our bodies heal.

Supplements

1. Mineral & Vitamin Supplements

Mineral supplements seem to be a very important addition to the diet for the typical person worth FMS. I have found an encapsulated form of mineral seems to be absorbed well into my body. When taking supplements, notice the effects they are having on your body. After a few days, I notice a definite increase in energy as well as a general over-all feeling of improved wellness. I feel it is important, if possible to have a medical practitioner or nutritionist help with a supplementation plan, although I have found that many are not as knowledgeable about FMS as they could be. I chose to use a supplementation that contains the ingredients necessary for a healthy body. The most important to help me feel better are: Manganese, Magnesium, Zinc, Malic Acid (for sleep). Iron, Calcium, Potassium, B-vitamins, Vitamin A, Copper, Vitamin E, Vitamin C and Bee Pollen.

Herbs

I love to grow parsley and eat 1-2 handfuls of it daily. When grown in your garden, parsley has a wonderful flavor and is full of vitamins and minerals, especially calcium.

Stretching Exercises

1. Eat at least one to one half hour before stretching (do not start on a full stomach).
2. These exercises are meant to be done very slowly and smoothly. Count to fifteen with each form before changing to a different exercise.
3. Begin taking three deep breaths before starting. Follow these steps for deep breathing:
   • Sit or stand tall noting the spinal chord being aligned and straight.
   • Begin to breath in through the nose filing the abdomen area first then the chest area.
   • Count to seven slowly while breathing in.
   • Breath out through the mouth to the count of seven, allowing air to leave the belly area first.
4. Slow, deep breaths should be taken during the exercises, exhaling on downward bends, inhaling on upward bends.
5. Each exercise should be held to a slow count of twenty. Remember the idea is to slowly stretch and strengthen, not to rush through the exercise. It should take approximately twenty minutes for each day's routine,
6. Pain is not the idea of these exercises. The "no pain no gain" rule does not apply here. Stretch to the point where you feel pulling. Stop and hold that point.
7. Use a soft, relaxing audio tape with either sounds of nature, instrumental music or piano music to keep the atmosphere relaxed. Many audio tapes are twenty minutes long, so they can act as a timer also.
8. Last, enjoy the beauty of the stretches and the flexibility it allows you to have.

• Often shoulders and upper back need more pressure than other parts of the body.
• A good massage therapist is a good source to stimulate the areas you are unable to reach. Family members or friends often are more than willing to help also.
• When doing the techniques, it is not necessary to do every technique in each section. Intended results can occur using as few as two or three of the points.
• Finally, enjoy using the acupressure techniques. As you learn the pressure points, this pain reducing technique will be something you can take with you wherever you go.

Stretching Exercise Plan #1

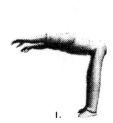 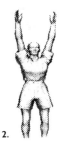 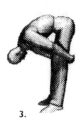

1. 2. 3.

1. Using the back of a chair or wall for support, bend at the waist stretching the back, shoulds and arm muscles. Count to twenty slowly, bend knees and stand up. Repeat this exercise three times.
2. While standing with feet shoulder width apart, move hands above head stretching the back, shoulders and arms. Breathe deeply, then let arms down. Repeat two times.
3. Bend at the waist and grasp hands behind the knees. Pull body close to the legs and hold to a slow count of twenty. Stand up and repeat exercise.

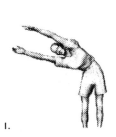 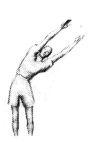 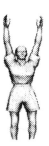

1. 2. 3.

1. With arms above the head as shown in picture #1, bend to the right. Count slowly to twenty.
2. With arms above the head as shown in picture #2, bend to the left, and count slowly to twenty.
3. With arms above the head, stretch the body up into the air as shown in picture #3.
4. Repeat all three exercises two times.

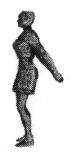 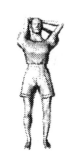 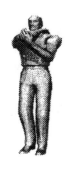

I.   **2.**   **3.**

1. While standing up straight, clasp hands behind the back. Breathe in slowly as the arms are lifted as shown in picture #1. Count slowly to twenty to release. Repeat.
2. Place right arm behind the head and with the right hand behind the head, grasp the right elbow with the left hand. Gently stretch the back muscles of the right arms while counting slowly to twenty. Repeat on the opposite side.
3. Bring the right hand over the front of the left shoulder. With the left hand, gently push the right elbow up towards the left shoulder. Hold to a slow count of twenty. Repeat on the opposite side.

Stretching Exercise Plan #2

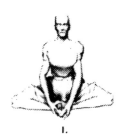 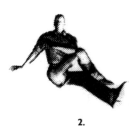 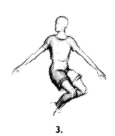

I.   **2.**   **3.**

1. While sitting on the floor bring the bottoms of the feet together. Place hands around the feet and gently pull the feet closer to your body. Count slowly to twenty and repeat exercise a second time.
2. Bring the right foot up over the left knee. Put the foot down flat against the floor as shown. Place the right hand on the floor behind you and bring the left hand over to hold the knee firmly. Count slowly to twenty. Repeat on the opposite side.
3. Lie on your back with arms out at the sides and heels against your buttocks. Roll knees over the right side so the left leg is on the floor. Count slowly to twenty and repeat exercise on the left side. Repeat two times.

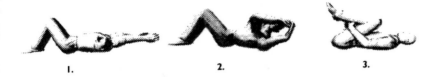

1. 2. 3.

1. Lie on your back with knees bent. Stretch arms above head while breathing deeply. Hold while counting to twenty slowly. Repeat two times.
2. Clasp hands and twist to the right as shown in the picture. Count slowly to twenty. Repeat exercise on opposite side. Repeat complete exercise two times.
3. Lie on your back and bend knees up onto abdomen. Count slowly to twenty. Repeat two times.

1. 2.

1. Lie on your stomach with forehead on the floor, place hands flat on the floor under shoulders. Count slowly to twenty.
2. With hands still under shoulders push up straightening the arms. Hold this position for a slow count of twenty. Repeat #1 and #2.

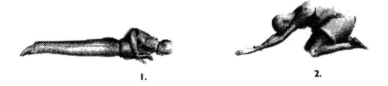

1. 2.

1. Lie on your stomach with forehead on the floor, placing hands flat on the floor under shoulders. Count slowly to twenty.
2. Place feet together and spread knees. With hands together, let the body drop down between the knees stretching arms out in front of the body. Let body relax down to the floor for two to four minutes. Repeat exercises #1 and #2.

Stretching Exercise Plan #3

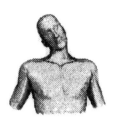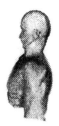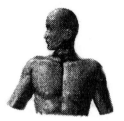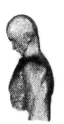

1. While standing or sitting up straight bend the head to the left as if to touch the left ear to the left shoulder. Count slowly to five. Repeat on the right side.
2. Bend the chin towards the neck, as if to make a double chin. Count to five slowly. Turn the head to the right, count slowly to five, then to the left. Count slowly to five.
3. Bend the head forward, then backward, counting slowly to five on each bend.

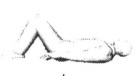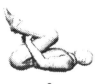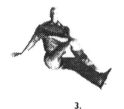

I. 2. 3.

1. While lying on the back, bring the legs up as in figure #1. Count slowly to twenty. Put legs down flat on to the floor. Breathe deeply two times.
2. Bring knees up onto abdomen, grasping hands under the knees. Count slowly to twenty.
3. Bring the right foot up over the left knee. Put the foot down flat against the floor as shown. Place the right hand on the floor behind you and bring the left hand over to hold the knee firmly. Countl slowly to twenty. Repeat on the opposite side.

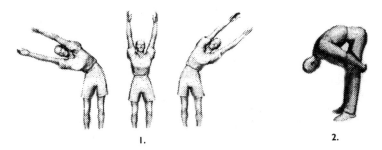

1.   2.

1. With arms above the head as shown, bend to the right. Count slowly to twenty. Move the hands above the head stretching the back, shoulders and arms. Breathe deeply, then let arms down. With arms above the head, bend to the left. Count slowly to twenty. Repeat exercise #1.

2. Bend at the waist and grasp hands behind the knees. Pull body close to the legs and hold to a slow count of twenty. Stand up and repeat exercise #2.

Acupressure Points

1. Deep breathing is very important to do to revitalize and purify the body. It is also important to deep breath before beginning the acupressure treatments to achieve optimum results.

2. Patients with life threatening illnesses or disease should always consult their doctor before using the accupressure or other alternative therapies. As I have mentioned in other areas of this book, all treatments in this book are treatments I've used on myself and my daughter for relief from the symptoms of FMS. This book is not intended as a substitute for medical advice from your physician. The reader should consult with his or her physician with any questions of health and/or symptoms that may require medical attention or diagnosis.

3. In doing acupressure on specific points, places a finger on the point and, without removing the finger, move it in three circular motions. Then gently press the area for one to three minutes.

4. The amount of pressure depends on the individual. If you experience pain, gently reduce pressure until you find a balance between pain and pleasure.

5. Acupressure is not intended to increase your tolerance for pain, discontinue pressing an area that is extremely painful.

6. Many times when you press on one point, you may feel pain in another part of the body. That pain indicates that those areas are related.

7. If your hands are in pain or too weak to use, knuckles, avocado pits, a golf ball or pencil eraser may be used to press on the points.

8. Shoulders and upper back will need more pressure than other parts of the body.

9. A good massage therapist can simulate areas you are not able to reach. My husband also tries to give me a firm back or foot massage two to four times per week, especially when I have tension and know my sleep will be affected by that tension.

10. Learn the points and their corresponding symptoms. You will then have a useful technique that will help control symptoms anytime they arise.

Headache or Neck-Head Pain Acupressure Points

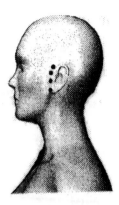 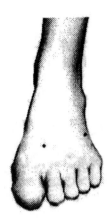

A. Location is one-half inch above the front of the depression in front of the ear which deepens when mouth is open.

B. Location is directly in front of the ear opening in a depression which deepens when mouth is open.

C.. Location is one-half inch below depression in B.

D. Location is the indention behind the earlobe.

E. Location at the top of the foot in the valley between the big toe and the second toe.

F. Located on top of the foot, one inch above the webbing of the fourth and fifth toes in the groove between the bones.

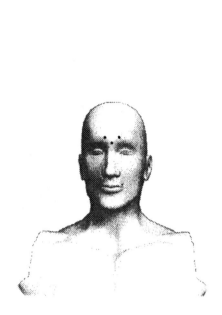
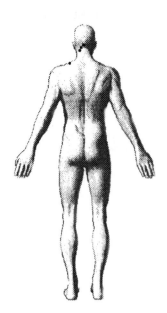

A. Location is in the indentations on either side of the bridge of the nose where the eyebrows meet the bridge of the nose.

B. Location is right in the middle where the bridge meets the forehead.

C. Location is at the bottom of the cheekbone, below the pupil of the eye.

D. Location in the center of the back of the head in a hollow under the base of the skull

E. Location is below the base of the skull between the two vertical neck muscles.

F. Located about one and one-half inches below the base of the skull, on the vertical muscles.

G. Located on the highest point of the shoulder muscle, one to two inches from the side of the lower neck. (Pregnant women should press this point lightly.)

Acupressure Points For Hip, Leg And Foot Pain

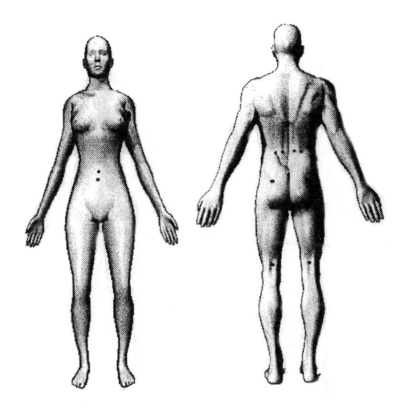

A.. Location is two finger widths directly below the belly button.
B. (Be sure not to press on any disintegrating disks or fractures or broken bones.) Located in the lower back, two finger widths away from the spine at the waist level.
C. Located in the lower back, four finger widths away from the spine at the waist level.
D. Located one to two finger widths out side the large bone in the base of the spine.
E. Located in the center of the back of the knee.

Acupressure Points For Shoulder, Arm, Hand, Middle and Upper Back Pain

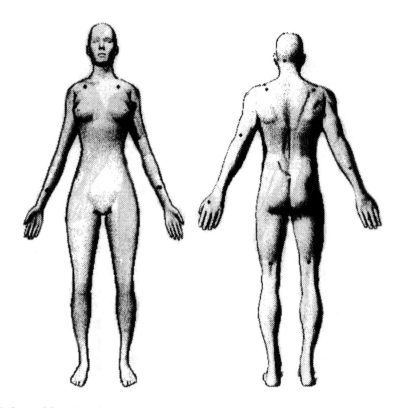

A. Located four finger-widths up from the armpit crease in the outer part of the chest, and one finger width inward.

B. Located on the inner wrist two and one-half finger widths up the arm from the center of the inner wrist.

C. Location is below the base of the skull between the two vertical neck muscle.

D. Located on the highest point of the shoulder muscle, one to two inches from the side of the lower neck. (pregnant women should press lightly on this point.).

E. Located one inch below and one-half inch to the center of D.

F.. Located in the center of the outer arm approximately one-third of the way down between the shoulder and the elbow where the upper arm muscle ends,

G. Located on the upper edge of the elbow crease.

H. Located two and one-half finger widths above the wrist crease on the outer forearm midway between the two bones of the arm.

I. Located in the webbing between the thumb and the index finger. (Pregnant women should not use this point.)

J. The waist points are located in the lower back two and four widths away from the spine at the waist level.

K. Located in the center of the back of the knee in the crease.

Acupressure Points For Immune System Booster

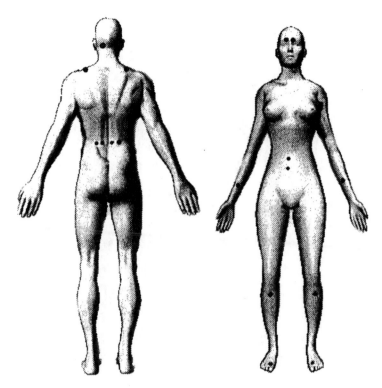

A. Location is below the base of the skull between the two vertical neck muscles.

B. Location is on the highest point on the shoulder muscle, one to two inches from the side of the lower neck.

C. Location in the lower back, two and four finger widths away from the spine at the waist level.

D. Location in the indentations on either side of the bridge of the nose where the eyebrows meet the bridge of the nose.

E. Two and one-half finger widths up the arm from the center of the inner wrist crease, midway between the two forearm bones.

F. Three fingers widths below the belly button.

G. Four fingers widths below the kneecap, and one finger width on the outside of the shin-bone. A muscle should flex as you move your feet up and down if you are on the right spot.

H. In the valley between the big toe and the second toe on the top of the feet.

Acupressure Points for Sleep

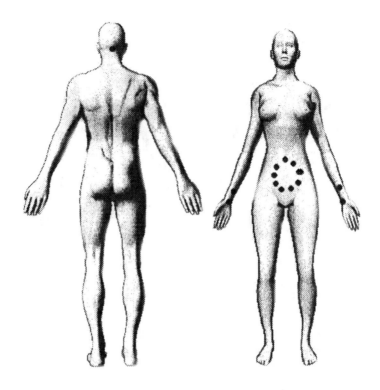

A. Location is in the center of the back of the head in a hollow under the base of the skull.

B. Located on the inner wrist two and one-half finger widths up the arm from the center of the inner wrist.

C. Located on the crease of the wrist toward the palm area of the hand.

D. Location begins four finger widths below the belly button. Continue at one o'clock, two o'clock, etc. around in a circle on the abdomen, pressing one inch inside of the hip bone structure and one inch above the pelvic bone.

APPENDIX

The Great Plains ☀ Laboratory (GPL)

For Health, Metabolism, and Nutrition

9335 W. 75 St.
Overland Park, Kansas 66204

Phone (913) 341-8949
Fax (913) 341-6207

Testing for yeast byproducts in the urine of fibromyalgia patients.

William Shaw Ph.D.

According to William Crook MD, the author of twelve books and numerous medical articles, "CFS/CFIDS and FMS are often yeast related . . .Increasing evidence shows that a sugar-free special diet and antifungal medications may help people with these chronic disorders get well." (1). At the Great Plains Laboratory, some of the reasons that yeast overgrowth causes so many problems are becoming clear. Below is a representative report of a urine sample from a patient with severe fibromyalgia. Note that there are four results flagged in the "high or H" category in the yeast/fungal section indicating values that exceed normal limits. The result for tartaric acid is most abnormal. The patient's value is 767 mmol/mol creatinine compared to a normal value of 16 mmol/mol creatinine. (All of these urine values are in terms of urine creatinine to compensate for differences in fluid intake.) **Thus, this value for tartaric acid is nearly 50 times that of normal!** In addition to the pain of fibromyalgia, this patient complains of depression and unclear thinking.

WHAT IS TARTARIC ACID AND WHAT IS IT DOING IN URINE? The main natural source of tartaric acid is yeast(2). This compound forms a sludge in the wine brewing process and has to be removed(2). Wine is sugar fermented by yeast to alcohol and other products. Humans do not produce this material. When yeast in the intestinal tract are fed sugar from the diet, they produce tartaric acid just like the yeast in the wine-making process. Why is tartaric acid harmful?

Tartaric acid is a muscle toxin and as little as 12 grams have been fatal to a human(3). One gram is about the weight of a cigarette. Tartaric acid is a muscle toxin and caused muscle damage when administered to experimental animals. Tartaric acid is also extremely elevated in many patients with fibromyalgia who also have muscle and joint pain. Tartaric acid was initially discovered by me in the urine of two autistic brothers with muscle weakness so severe that they could not stand up(4).

Tartaric acid is an analog (a close chemical relative) of malic acid (Figure 1). Malic acid is a key intermediate in the Krebs cycle, a biochemical process used for the extraction of most of the energy from our food. Presumably tartaric acid is toxic because it inhibits the biochemical production of the normal compound, malic acid. Tartaric acid is a known inhibitor of the Krebs cycle enzyme fumarase (Figure 2), which produces malic acid from fumaric acid(5). A large percentage of patients with fibromyalgia respond favorably to treatment with malic acid(6). I presume that supplements of malic acid are able to overcome the toxic effects of tartaric acid by supplying deficient malic acid. Treatment with the antifungal drug Nystatin kills the yeast and values for tartaric acid steadily diminish with antifungal treatment (Figure 3). Fifty percent of patients with fibromyalgia often suffer from hypoglycemia(7)(low blood sugar) even though their diet may have adequate or even excessive sugar. The reason may be due to the inhibition of the Krebs cycle by tartaric acid. The Krebs cycle is the main provider of raw material such as malic acid that can be converted to blood sugar(Figure 2) when the body uses up its supply. If sufficient malic acid cannot be produced, the body cannot produce the sugar glucose which is the main fuel for the brain. The person with hypoglycemia feels weak and their thinking is foggy because there is insufficient fuel for their brain.

WHERE IS THIS YEAST AND WHY DO I HAVE THIS PROBLEM? Most of the time the yeast are present only in the intestinal tract, not in the blood and other organs. However, the tartaric acid and other compounds produced by yeast in the intestine are absorbed into the bloodstream and may enter all of the cells of the body. Dr. St Anand noticed that patients with fibromyalgia had high amounts of dental tartar on their teeth and speculated that similar deposits in the muscles and ligaments might be causing the pain of fibromyalgia. I suspect that tartaric acid is the compound found in the dental tartar and that crystals of this substance may be causing the muscle and joint pain just as kidney stones cause kidney pain. The two main causes of yeast overgrowth are use of broad-spectrum antibiotics and the high sugar and carbohydrate diet of American diet. Broad spectrum antibiotics kill most of the normal bacteria(germs) in the intestinal tract but do not kill organisms such as yeast (8-15). As a matter of fact, some yeast grow faster in the presence of antibiotics. The reason fibromyalgia commonly follows traumatic accidents may be related to the use of antibiotics to treat trauma. Sugar consumption is the second major factor in causing yeast related illnesses. The average American consumes 10 times more sugar (about 150 lb per year) than Americans in the time of George Washington. In a study done in mice, mice receiving sugar in their water had 200 times more yeast in their intestine than mice receiving plain water(16). Other factors that cause yeast over-growth may include stress, birth control pills, viral infections, and a weak immune system(Figure 4).

WHAT CAN I DO ABOUT THIS PROBLEM IF I HAVE IT? The yeast problem can be treated with a combination of low sugar, low carbohydrate diet, an antifungal drug to kill the yeast, and probiotics, which are supplements of *Lactobacillus acidophilus* to restore beneficial bacteria to the intestinal tract. Malic acid and magnesium supplements will help the patient until the yeast problem is resolved which may be about two months. The reduction of tartaric acid in urine following antifungal treatment is illustrated in Figure 3.

HOW DO I GET THE TEST DONE? A medical practitioner who is licensed to order urine testing in your state must approve the test order. Regulations vary from state to state so an approved medical practitioner could be a medical doctor(MD), osteo-path(DO), nurse practitioner, chiropractor(DC), or naturopath(ND). If you have any difficulty in getting your physician to approve the test, we can refer you to a suitable physician in most locations in the United States and in some foreign countries. The test is reimbursed by most insurance companies but we cannot guarantee reimbursement. A morning urine sample is shipped to The Great Plains Laboratory and results are usually available in 48-72 hours with a recommendation to your physician for treatment.

WHAT OTHER INFORMATION WILL I GET FROM YOUR TEST? The test evaluates all of the well-defined inborn errors of metabolism that can be detected with this technology called GCIMS such as PKU, maple-syrup urine disease, and many others. In addition, I check for many other abnormalities such as vitamin deficiencies and abnormal metabolism of catecholamines, dopamine, and serotonin. We currently quantitate 62 substances but also evaluate other substances that are not quantitated. For example, in the sample report, high kynurenic acid indicated a need for vitamin B-6 and the evaluated glutaric acid indicated a requirement for coenzyme Q10. Even if you don't have the yeast problem, your test may still be beneficial to you.

I HAVE AN HMO AND THEY HAVE TO SEND THE TEST TO A CERTAIN LAB, IS THAT OK?
No. No other laboratory routinely analyzes the same compounds as this laboratory including Labcorp, Smithkline, or Mayo Medical laboratories. If you do not specify our laboratory, your urine will be sent to one of the large reference labs which cannot accurately evaluate your condition. Most test for the inborn errors of metabolism and that's all.

WHAT ABOUT REIMBURSEMENT FOR MEDICAID AND MEDICARE? We are now set up for Medicare but we do not yet have Medicaid authorization.

WILL DRUGS OR ANY OF THESE NUTRITIONAL SUPPLEMENTS INTERFERE IN THE ORGANIC ACID TEST? No, there is no interference from any known drug or supplement. However, if antifungal supplements or drugs are taken before the test, you will probably get a lower value for the yeast byproducts. I advise you to get the test first so that you will know what the starting point is. The malic acid and magnesium products will not affect the test results.

I DON'T HAVE INSURANCE AND CAN'T AFFORD THE PRICE. CAN YOU HELP ME? We would be happy to work out an installment plan for you. Mastercard and VISA payments are also acceptable.

I HAVE BEEN DISABLED DUE TO THE SEVERITY OF MY FIBROMYALGIA YET HAVE NOT BEEN ABLE TO GET BENEFITS. COULD THIS TEST HELP ME TO GET BENEFITS? This test could benefit you if we document a defined biochemical disorder. Of greater importance is the possibility of reversing the fibromyalgia if the yeast problem is a significant factor.

WHAT CAN I DO IF MY PHYSICIAN DOESN'T UNDERSTAND THE TEST RESULTS? I will be glad to help you and your physician develop a suitable therapy based on your individual test results.

MY DOCTOR SAYS EVERYONE HAS YEAST IN THEIR INTESTINE AND IF YEAST WERE THE CAUSE OF FIBROMYALGIA THEN EVERYONE WOULD BE ADVERSELY AFFECTED. HOW DO ANSWER THAT ASSERTION? The most important question is not whether yeast are present or not. The critical factors are the quantity of yeast and the kinds and amounts of toxic products they produce. Everyone in this society has carbon monoxide in their blood and can tolerate a low value. When the amount of carbon monoxide increases, some individuals feel depressed, some have headaches, some develop muscle weakness, some feel tightness in the chest or angina, some experience nausea and vomiting, some become dizzy, some develop dimming of vision. As values increase, symptoms may include convulsions, coma, respiratory failure, and death. Individuals who recover from severe carbon monoxide poisoning may suffer residual neurological damage. Different people will respond with different symptoms to the same concentration of carbon monoxide. Why is it surprising that exposure to a wide range of toxic yeast products at different times and at different ages might produce different symptoms? If I suggested that there were a carbon monoxide connection with all of the diverse symptoms associated with carbon monoxide exposure, no one would challenge me. The reason that the carbon monoxide connection is accepted is because carbon monoxide can be easily measured in blood. The toxic yeast products were just discovered but as knowledge of them increases, acceptance of the yeast related illnesses will increase. The philosopher Schopenhauer said "All truth goes through three stages. First, it is ridiculed. Then, it is violently opposed. Finally, it is accepted as self-evident." Within five years, people who ignore the importance of yeast related illness will be in the same camp with those in the Flat-Earth Society.

QUOTED FROM SIDNEY MACDONALD BAKER MD IN THE BOOK *DETOXIFICATION AND HEALING, THE KEY TO OPTIMAL HEALTH*: "Dr Shaw's work is very recent and as I write this he has just opened a new lab.. The reason for telling you about his work is to ask you to think about the implications and watch as his ideas develop over the next few years. As you will see in the next chapter, there is other evidence to support these ideas and, if you understand the implications, there are things you can do now that will reduce your risk of ill health while continuing to watch from the sidelines." Dr. Baker is a graduate of Yale University School of Medicine and is board certified in obstetrics and pediatrics. Dr. Baker was director of the Gessell Institute of Human Development and has taught at Yale Medical School and is the author of dozens of articles and several books about health and nutritional biochemistry.

References

1. Crook William, The Yeast Connection Handbook. Jackson, TN, 1997:34-35.
2. Tartaric acid. Microsoft Encarta 96 Encyclopedia on CD ROM.
3. Webster R. Legal Medicine and Toxicology. WB Saunders, Philadelphia, 1930:413-414.
4. Shaw W. Kassen E, and Chaves E. Increased excretion of analogs of Krebs cycle metabolites and arabinose in two brothers with autistic features. Clinical Chemistry 41:1094-1104,1995.
5. Mahler H and Cordes. Biological Chemistry. New York, Harper and Row. 1966:417-418.
6. Holzschlag Molly. CoQ1O, malic acid, and magnesium may improve CFIDSIFM symptoms. The CFIDS Chronicle, Summer 1993.
7. St Amand RP. Exploring the fib romyalgia connection. The Vulvar Pain Newslet-ter. Fall 1996,4-6.
8. Kennedy M and Volz P Dissemination of yeasts after gastrointestinal inoculation in antibiotic-treated mice. Sabouradia 21:27-33,1983.
9. Danna P, Urban C, Bellin E, and Rahal J. Role of Candida in pathogenesis of antibiotic associated diarrhoea in elderly patients. Lancet 337:511-14, 1991.
10. Osfleld E, Rubinstein E, Gazit E, Smetana Z. Effect of systemic antibiotics on the microbial flora of the external ear canal in hospitalized children. Pediat 60:364-66,1977.
11. Kinsman OS, Pitblado K. Cand ida albicans gastrointestinal colonization and invasion in the mouse: effect of antibacterial dosing, antifungal therapy, and immunosuppression. Mycoses 32:664-74, 1989.
12. Van der Waaij D. Colonization resistance of the digestive tract-mechanism and clinical consequences. Nahrung 31:507-17,1987.
13. Samonis G and Dassiou M. Antibiotics affecting gastrointestinal colonization of mice by yeasts. Chemotherapy 6: 50-2,1994.
14. Samonis G., Gikas A, and Toloudis, P. Prospective evaluation of the impact of broad-spectrum antibiotics on the yeast flora of the human gut. Euro Jour of Clin Micro Infec Dis, 13(1994): 665-67.
15. Samonis G, Gikas A, and Anaissie E. Prospective evaluation of the impact of broad-spectrum antibiotics on gastrointestinal yeast colonization of humans. Antimicrobian agens and Chemotherapy 37(1993): 51-53.
16. Vargas S, Patrick C, Ayers G, and Hughes W. Modulating effect of dietary carbohydrate supplementation on Candida albicans colonization and invasion in a neutropenic mouse model. Infection and Immunity 61(1993): 619-626.

The Great Plains Laboratory

9335 W. 75 St.
Overland Park, Kansas 66204

Phone (913) 341-8949
Fax (913) 341-6207

CLIA ID# 17D0919496
William Shaw, Ph.D., Laboratory Director

Patient Name	Jane Doe		Date of Collection	2/11/97
Patient Age	36		Time of Collection	8:50 AM
Physician Name	John Smith, M.D.		Patient Sex	Female

Name	mmol/mol creatinine		Reference range mmol/mol creatinine	Name	mmol/mol creatinine		Reference range mmol/mol creatinine
Glycolysis				**Yeast/Fungal**			
lactic	22.15		0-100	citramalic	4.42	H	0-2
pyruvic	9.82		0-50	5-hydroxymethyl-2-furoic	98	H	0-80
2-hydroxybutyric	1.06		0-2	3-oxoglutaric	0.46		0-0.5
glyceric	8.17		0-10	furan-2,5-dicarboxylic	67.01	H	0-50
Amino Acid Metabolites				furancarbonylglycine	0		0-60
2-hydroxyisovaleric	0.10		0-2	tartaric	767	H	0-16
2-oxoisovaleric	0.19		0-2	arabinose	27		0-115
3-methyl-2-oxovaleric	0.24		0-2	carboxycitric	0.81		0-46
hydroxyisocaproic	0.02		0-2	**Bacterial**			
2-oxoisocaproic	0.23		0-2	2-hydroxyphenylacetic	0.61		0-10
2-oxo-4-methiolbutyric	0.03		0-2	4-hydroxyphenylacetic	41		0-50
mandelic	0.31		0-5	**Anaerobic Bacterial**			
phenyllactic	0.24		0-2	DHPPA analog	103		0-150
phenylpyruvic	0.14		0-5	VMA analog	15.41		0-31
homogentisic	0.87		0-2	**Krebs Cycle**			
4-hydroxyphenyllactic	2		0-50	succinic	3		0-20
pyroglutamic	9	L	20-115	fumaric	1.31		0-10
3-indoleacetic	8.68		0-10	2-oxo-glutaric	29.57		15-200
kynurenic	2.82	H	0-2	aconitic	35	H	0-25
Fatty Acid Metabolites				citric	23		20-200
3-hydroxybutyric	0.78		0-10	**Neurotransmitters**			
acetoacetic	17.12	H	0-10	HVA	16.53		0-25
ethylmalonic	0.08		0-10	VMA	3.23		0-18
methylsuccinic	2.68		0-5	5-hydroxyindoleacetic	1.08		0-20
adipic	6.41		0-12	**Pyrimidines**			
suberic	3.67	H	0-2	uracil	11.96		0-22
sebacic	1.28		0-2	thymine	0.33		0-2
Miscellaneous				**Miscellaneous**			
glutaric	2.21	H	0-2	glycolic	57		0-100
methylmalonic	1.09		0-5	oxalic	17.06		0-100
N-acetyl aspartic	8.44		0-100	malonic	0.20		0-10
ascorbic	8501.43	H	10-200	methylglutaric	0.89		0-10
orotic	0.06		0-3.5	hippuric	677	H	10-400
3-hydroxy-3-methylglutaric	3.31		0-36	4-hydroxybutyric	2.34		0-5
hydroxyhippuric	2.08		0-20	phenylcarboxylic	0.21		0-15
				indole-like compound	9.56		0-60

Figure 1. Comparison of chemical structure of malic and tartaric acid. Differences shaded in gray.

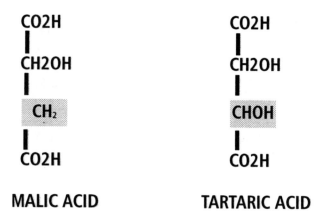

Figure 2. Site of tartaric acid inhibition of Krebs cycle, the major energy producing mechanism of the cell. In addition to the inhibition of energy production, tartaric acid prevents the production of malic acid, which is a key intermediate in the production of glucose in the process of gluconeogenesis, the principal fuel for the brain.

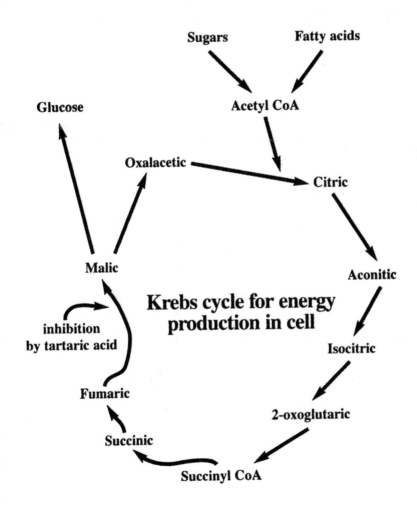

Figure 3. Patient with high tartaric acid was started on the antifungal drug Nystatin and then tested while on this drug. Even after 68 days, tartaric increased when the dose was reduced in half and then decreased again when the full dose of antifungal drug was restored.

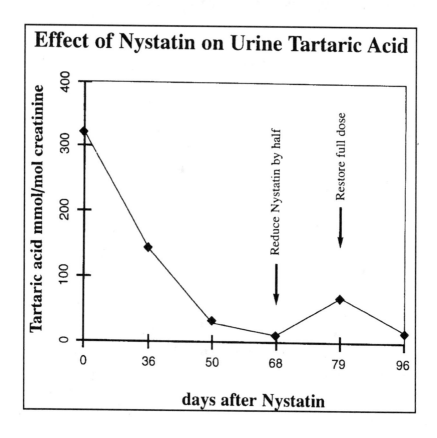

Figure 4. Factors contributing to yeast overgrowth in fibromyalgia.

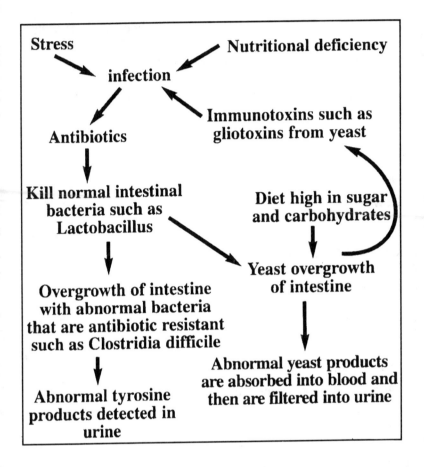

This book has been donated to your public library by Fibromyalgia Solutions

For recipes look for The Fibromyalgia Nutrition Guide written by Mary Moeller & Dr. Joe Elrod or visit Mary's web site at www.fibrosolutions.com. (If you don't have access to the internet, ask your librarian for help)

Other books Mary has written on Fibromyalgia include:

Fibromyalgia, Beginning the Road to Health *Booklet with stories of others who have or are recovering & info on symptoms and nutritional deficiencies* $3.95 Available at Health Food Stores

Overcoming Fibromyalgia, A Guide For Recovery *Three month daily guide which includes recipes, information on sugars and flours, candida questionnaire, exercise program, information on the sleep cycle and natural ways to help get a better nights sleep and pain control.* $14.95 Available at most major book stores.

The Fibromyalgia Nutrition Guide Written by Mary Moeller and Dr. Joe Elrod *Recipe book* $14.95 Available at most book stores.

Visit our web site at www.fibrosolutions.com to order the above books and other products. Visit our web site for more information on fibromyalgia and chronic fatigue syndrome, other recipes and answers to frequently asked questions and more.

If you would like to have Mary come to your church or organization to speak on fibromyalgia or to give a motivational presentation, she may be contacted by calling toll free 888-743-4276 or 816-903-5427 (Kansas City area).

...naturally.
...her
...ges includ-
grams and
while

A ...
Th...
da...
in...
a ...
de...

To...
Fi...
FM...

Fil...

FM...

M...

Yo...

Total Cost

...rs Accepted